KEY DEBATES IN SOCIAL WORK AND PHILOSOPHY

In order to practise effectively in today's complex and changing environment, social workers need to have an understanding of how contemporary cultural and philosophical concepts relate to the people they work with and the fields they practise in. Exploring the ideas of philosophers, including Nietzsche, Gadamer, Taylor, Adorno, MacIntyre, Žižek and Derrida, this text demonstrates their relevance to social work practice and presents new approaches and frameworks to understanding social change.

Key Debates in Social Work and Philosophy introduces a range of concerns central to social work and social care, with chapters looking at questions such as:

- What is the 'self'?
- How are communities formed?
- Why is 'choice' important?
- Are certain rights really applicable to all humans?
- What are the political and ethical implications of documenting your practice?
- What does it mean to be a professional social worker?

Each chapter focuses on a particular area of dispute, presenting the relevant philosophical theories, and considering how social work examples and research can be used to inform theoretical debate. Each chapter includes questions to prompt discussion and reflection.

The only book to examine the philosophical ideas that underlie and inform contemporary issues for social work and social care practitioners, this is a useful resource for those studying social work theory, policy and practice.

Tom Grimwood is Senior Lecturer and Programme Lead for the MA Social Work programme at the University of Cumbria, UK.

KEY DEBATES IN SOCIAL WORK AND PHILOSOPHY

Tom Grimwood

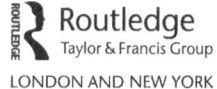
LONDON AND NEW YORK

First published 2016
by Routledge
2 Park Square, Milton Park, Abingdon, Oxon OX14 4RN

and by Routledge
711 Third Avenue, New York, NY 10017

Routledge is an imprint of the Taylor & Francis Group, an informa business

© 2016 T. Grimwood

The right of Tom Grimwood to be identified as author of this work has been asserted by him in accordance with sections 77 and 78 of the Copyright, Designs and Patents Act 1988.

All rights reserved. No part of this book may be reprinted or reproduced or utilised in any form or by any electronic, mechanical, or other means, now known or hereafter invented, including photocopying and recording, or in any information storage or retrieval system, without permission in writing from the publishers.

Trademark notice: Product or corporate names may be trademarks or registered trademarks, and are used only for identification and explanation without intent to infringe.

British Library Cataloguing-in-Publication Data
A catalogue record for this book is available from the British Library

Library of Congress Cataloging in Publication Data
Grimwood, Tom (Thomas David), author.
Key debates in social work and philosophy / Tom Grimwood.
p. ; cm.
Includes bibliographical references and index.
I. Title.
[DNLM: 1. Social Work–ethics. 2. Philosophy. HV 40]
R724
174.2–dc23
2015015912

ISBN: 978-0-415-74453-9 (hbk)
ISBN: 978-0-415-74454-6 (pbk)
ISBN: 978-1-315-81299-1 (ebk)

Typeset in Bembo
by Cenveo Publisher Services
Printed by Ashford Colour Press Ltd, Gosport, Hants

For Paul Fletcher, who would have probably disagreed.

CONTENTS

Preface ix

Introduction: Why should social workers think about philosophy, and why should philosophers care? 1

1 Interpretation: Social work and hermeneutics 14

2 Community: The case of the missing community 36

3 Identity: A short word from Nietzsche: marginalisation, recognition and *ressentiment* 60

4 Ethics: Three concerns about human rights 81

5 Documents: The politics of writing 105

6 Self: Who am I, and what do I actually do? 127

7 Culture: The culture industry 151

8 Knowledge: Professionalised practice and the locus of expertise 172

Index 191

PREFACE

In the early stages of my career, I taught philosophy and cultural theory within humanities departments, mainly delivering modules that explored how interpretation, ethics and social practices all engaged one another. At some point in my career, the students in the classroom changed from philosophy students to social work students. The modules changed – the social practices were now defined more specifically, particular to social work – but the explorations remained, in a modified form. And while I would never claim that these are the modules social work students always really *want* to do – suffice to say, Paul Michael Garrett's short story about his student who declares that social theory won't 'get you through the door' has been reproduced in my classroom on numerous occasions – I am always struck by how often the topics and discussions intersect closely with those of my earlier philosophy courses. Despite the emphasis on the social and natural sciences within social work's educational frameworks in the United Kingdom, the philosophical questions that emerge within every aspect of social work education and scholarship are unavoidable. And the discussions that such questions lead to are, in many cases, good philosophical ones. And thus, an idea for a book was born: not on the 'philosophy of social work' directly, but rather a book about the intersections and resonances between the two disciplines that will, I hope, be of interest to a social work audience.

As with any book, this would not have actually been written without the support, guidance and encouragement of many interlocutors over many years, although some will certainly not have known that they were offering it at the time. In particular, I would like to thank Grace McInnes, Rebecca Pearce and Louisa Vahtrick at Routledge, as well as the anonymous reviewers of the initial proposal, my colleagues in the Social Work team at the University of Cumbria, the speakers and organisers of the UoC Arts Research Initiative, Paul Fletcher, Stephen Gibbs, Sarah

Hitchen, Gavin Hyman, Martin Lang, Hugh McLaughlin, Shuruq Naguib, Alison Scott-Bauman, Naomi Sharples, Alison Stone, and, in particular, Arthur Bradley. Conversations with Rhona O'Brien helped to make connections between theory and practice I wouldn't have otherwise made; Carol Travers and Vicki Goodwin both provided timely and much needed sounding boards throughout the project; and my ongoing arguments (and erstwhile collaborations) with Paul Miller continue to drive much of my research.

Finally, and most importantly, the work would have been utterly impossible without the endless patience of Abby, and the endless distractions of Elijah.

INTRODUCTION

Why should social workers think about philosophy, and why should philosophers care?

Thinking at the intersections

For some, the intersection between philosophy and social work needs little justification. As Mel Gray and Stephen Webb write, 'to "think social work" is to engage with and against contemporary and past theorists and theoretical concepts', which will almost inevitably involve crossing philosophical paths. Such crossing of paths is fundamental, as the 'joy of "thinking social work" is in creating alternative modes of understanding through critical engagement with competing perspectives' (Gray and Webb 2013: 7). Likewise, Gianni Vattimo and Santiago Zabala argue that 'philosophy is not a disengaged, contemplative, or neutral reception of objects but rather the practice of an interested, projected, and active possibility' (2011: 14).

However, a common reaction to the idea of 'doing philosophy' on a social work course is a combative one: from the dismissive 'what's that got to do with social work?' to the hostile 'social work is about practice, not idealistic theories brought out from ivory towers!', and a whole range in between. While it is true these may only reflect clichés of what both social work and philosophy actually are, it is equally true that clichés emerge through the frequency and repetition of their use, and nowhere is this more evident than the crude caricatures of 'theory' and 'practice' that have often dominated social work as a discipline. What Chris Jones has termed the 'anti-intellectual tradition' in social work has by now been both well-documented and well-criticised. Indeed, the space for in-depth 'theoretical' discussion within pre-registration social work programmes has often been limited by the perception that it competes with the 'practical' skills-based work of qualificatory education; a perception often shared not only between students but also between government policy-makers (see Garrett 2013: 214). While social work practice only ever takes place within some kind of theoretical framework, whether acknowledged or not (Coulshed and Orme 2006), social workers can nevertheless 'turn cold' at the introduction of what they view as 'esoteric, abstract, and something people discuss in universities' (Mullaly 1997: 99). Jones notes the 'specific and utilitarian manner' in which mainstream social work has approached social research in the United Kingdom: 'theories, perspectives, insights and research findings are plundered', but rarely 'in a spirit of genuine intellectual inquiry or exploration' (Jones 1996: 194). Despite the development of both Bachelor's and Master's degree programmes for social work qualification, there remains in many areas an affirmation of the atheoretical as a mark of professional virtue (Mullaly 1997: 100). The effectiveness of the theory/practice cliché is testified to by the fact that exactly this kind of opening paragraph can be seen in the introductions to almost every available book on social work theory.

Of course, such provisos are given in order to be contested. In Gray and Webb's words, 'social work practice is the bearer and articulation of more or less theory-laden beliefs and concepts. Even those who… [claim] that social work is just "good common sense" are, in fact, articulating a distilled version of philosophical theories about common sense' (Gray and Webb 2013: 5). Research has often shown that social workers rarely use 'theory' in formal or explicit ways (see Fook 2000). They can often utilise theories without identifying or naming them (Howe 1987), but nevertheless draw meaningful sense from complex situations. In this way social workers are always theorising in some shape or form. Indeed, relatively straightforward activities such as interpreting communicative cues, identifying individual agency, assessing actions and promoting freedoms, can only be carried out on the basis of fundamental philosophical commitments regarding how meaning is created, what a self is, why agency is important, the nature of the 'good', and so on.

If this is the case with social work's view of philosophy, then what about the return match – why don't philosophers talk about social work? There is a range of answers to this, and, just as before, we must be careful not to fall prey to glib generalisations or stereotypes regarding the purpose of the discipline. After all, as Josef Niźnik has noted, the idea that philosophy is somehow intrinsically divorced from questions of social need, marginalisation or power is not borne out by its history:

> Reflection on the social context of human life appeared together with the human capacity to think about oneself, a capacity marking the beginnings of philosophy. The problems of the social conditions of man, and of institutions such as the state or of such values as justice, occupied a place in the repertoire of problems dealt with by the first philosophers as important as that of ontological or cosmological questions. (Niźnik 2006: 90)

The applied social sciences do not hold exclusive rights to concerns for the social world. Perhaps rather too often, this is obscured by the relationship between philosophy and the social sciences being figured as somewhat hierarchical – philosophy handles the 'big' ideas, while social sciences deal with the individual cases that make up the big ideas – rather than a two-way conversation between concepts and their application (see Grimwood and Miller 2014). Of course, in order to provide an encompassing philosophical argument regarding the world of human interaction, *some* level of abstraction seems necessary to render the argument meaningful: not because of the demands of any formal argumentation, but rather as an important (and pragmatic) link between particular cases and their more general application. As early as the late second century CE, Hermagoras of Temnos (Lanham 1991: 150) identified this as the difference between a *hypothesis* and a *thesis*: specific or empirical events (the hypotheses) are rendered meaningful within an overarching framework (the thesis). Thus, despite the visible prominence of its younger 'rivals' such as sociology and psychology within social work curricula, philosophy nevertheless continues to underpin their theories and ground their methods. As Niźnik comments, there is no need to see philosophical concerns as substitutes or antagonists of sociological or psychological ones. They not only display 'the variety of methodological concepts, languages and doctrines familiar from philosophy, but […] [t]hey are also close to one another in so far as they respond to the human need for understanding' (2006: 89–90).

But aren't they different types of reasoning?

Nevertheless, there may well be a *philosophical* objection to bridging the two disciplines, which is worth considering at this point. A version of this objection can be found in the influential essay by Immanuel Kant, 'An Answer to the Question: "What is Enlightenment?"', written in 1784. Here, Kant laid out what can be seen as an effective manifesto for modern philosophy, based on the principles of enlightenment. This involves, it could be argued, a separation of philosophical thinking from what can be interpreted as practice-based thinking. 'Enlightenment', Kant begins, 'is man's emergence from his self-incurred immaturity. Immaturity is the inability to use one's own understanding without the guidance of another. This immaturity is self-incurred if its cause is not lack of understanding, but lack of resolution and courage to use it without the guidance of another' (Kant 1996: 11). We need to think for ourselves, and not on the unquestioned basis of what others tell us (be they lecturers, practice educators, government policies or whatever), or on the basis of 'just what's done around here'.

But this obviously does not mean we do as we please; as that could hardly count as intellectual maturity. In pursuing our newly-found maturity, it is necessary to distinguish between the application of reasoning that is 'courageous', and reasoning that simply lets us get on with our lives. Thus, for Kant, we exercise a *private reason* when doing our jobs during the day, and a *public reason* in our reflective time after the shift is through. We may, Kant suggests, work in a tax office during the day, and utilise a certain rational way of thinking in order to do the job well (ordering the files, employing mathematical models, etc.). But our *philosophical* reasoning emerges when we go home at night, and write letters to the newspapers arguing how unfair the tax system is as a whole. Nearly 250 years after Kant put forward this argument, it would still not be an unfamiliar picture to imagine social workers conducting their assessments and interventions for social services departments during the day, but questioning after hours whether they were empowering individuals or merely acting as agents of the state. Jobs, according to Kant, require *private* reasoning because such thinking only extends as far as helping us as individuals play out our occupational role – to be, in Kant's words, 'a cog in a machine'. While such instrumental reasoning may still come under the remit of philosophy (there are good and bad ways to do a job, after all), this is ultimately secondary to the consideration of the ends which instrumental reasoning aims at. Hence, *public* reasoning requires us to think beyond our own individual circumstance and consider society, and the world, as a whole. It asks about the role and purpose of the job in the wider scheme of things. When we do this, we are reasoning as a rational being, rather than a cog in a machine: 'when one is reasoning as a member of reasonable humanity, then the use of reason must be free and public' (Foucault 1984: 37). To be fully 'public', of course, the concern of reason for reason's sake must be *universal* rather than *contextual*. Hence, for Kant, philosophers might be interested in discussing questions such as whether we should *always* obey the law, even if that law conflicts with our values; whereas, for social workers, there are rather more pressing requirements to follow legal procedures determined by the context of their jobs. Public reason is necessary for society to reach enlightened 'maturity', whilst private reason is essential for there to be a society in the first place. And if the two are distinct, then it seems only natural for social workers to flip the argument around and ask: 'how does thinking about concepts and causes really help me to do my job in the *here and now*?'

This separation between the kind of thinking that enables us to do a predefined job, with a clear set of aims and objectives, and the kind of thinking that is more typically seen as 'philosophical', could be said to have informed a distinction within the work of philosophy itself. Textbooks on philosophical ethics will frequently point out that while professions rely on ethical codes, these are not really the subject of philosophy: they are, instead, simply rules to follow. For example, Alex Barber suggests that courses on vocational ethics 'sometimes contain elements of moral philosophy', but more commonly 'they aim merely at presenting a list of professional protocols, i.e. rules for proper conduct in the relevant domain' (2010: 8). Or, as Andrew Alexandra and Seumas Miller state in their philosophical discussion of professional ethics: 'That professionals have a range of special duties (and rights) seems undeniable […]. The question we address here is: "Where do these duties come from?"' (2009: 104). The difference between the two seems to stem both from the manner in which they are learned – philosophical ethics are, generally speaking, more 'up for discussion' in the classroom than professional ethics, at least at most levels – and a broader debate within the history of philosophy, to which Kant's argument was one decisive contributor: the debate over the kinds of thinking we do, and the relationship between these kinds of thinking and the distinctive activities that comprise different realms of human existence – work, play, family, etc.

This distinction, however, has long been debated within social work itself. Social work education as a whole sits within such a contested dialectical relationship between 'field education' or 'practice placements' and classroom-based questioning, analysis and reflection; or, between 'training' for the technical, day-to-day aspects of the job, and 'education' for a broader understanding of the potentially transformative role of the social worker within society. Donald Schön famously critiqued the notion of practice as a form of 'technical rationality' where 'practitioners are instrumental problem solvers, who select technical means best suited to particular purposes' (1987: 3); Neil Thompson has frequently advocated a 'dialectical relationship' between theory and practice (2010: 15). Hence, it is important to question Kant's distinction itself on several grounds, which in turn help to articulate how the relationship between the disciplines of social work and philosophy should be considered.

Challenging dichotomies, clarifying relationships

First, it is important to remember that Kant's argument is brief: a manifesto, in a sense, of the kind of thinking he associated with the prospective new age of Enlightenment. Instrumental reason might be utilised in order to get the job done, but this is all premised on the *right job* being done, which accorded to the principles of Enlightenment itself. In this sense, instrumental reason is not *opposed* to speculative thinking. Kant himself famously argued that 'thoughts without content are empty, intuitions without concepts are blind' (Kant 1993: 69). There is, in fact, a clear lineage between the kind of moral society envisaged by Kant that was, via the work of Fichte, subsequently applied to social contexts in the work of British philosopher T.H. Green, and the work of the early forms of social work practice – most notably, the Charity Organisation Society and the Settlement House Movement in the United Kingdom and the United States – which were heavily influenced by these ideas (see Simon 1994; Lewis 1995; Pierson 2011).

Second, if this underpinning of the early forms of social work has since dissipated, the 'work' of social work must nevertheless be conceived broadly. As Hugman argues, it is confined neither to the micro-level of individual small-scale change, nor to the macro-level of structural development: 'It is about both of these things, sometimes separately and sometimes together. In short, social work is about the personal *and* the political' (Hugman 2013: 159, my emphasis). This suggests that the practicalities of social work go beyond instrumental reason alone. This has been clear since at least Plant's 1970 work *Social and Moral Theory in Casework*, which was one of the first texts to explore the philosophical depth of the day-to-day tasks of social work. And since Plant's work, the idea of there even being a unified 'method' of social work has fragmented amongst a complex history of antagonistic relationships between competing models, approaches, directives and organisation. Consequently, the very question of where to draw the line between instrumental and normative reasoning is itself a philosophical discussion that social work is inherently part of; consider, for example, debates such as the criticisms of task-centred practice as prioritising an individualist sense of 'getting the job done', over and above broader issues of social and economic relationships (see Dominelli 1996). It is the practice of philosophy, I think, to track the modes of thought which link these otherwise separate areas together – personal and political, individual and social, and so on –

and to unpack the conditions of such connections and disconnections that lie within them.

This is why to simply perceive philosophy as something other-worldly and distinct from the day-to-day practical tasks of social work is a mistake. In part, this is because the *time* and *space* available for bringing to the fore of our everyday activities their philosophical content is often limited to distinct and separate spaces, and often such a space is, indeed, as 'other-worldly' as a university classroom or quiet supervision behind closed doors. The space where we *articulate* the philosophical dimension of social work is often not the space where it actually *happens*. True, much philosophy may appear to be abstract and therefore difficult, initially, to relate to the day-to-day tasks of practice. But this does not separate the impact they have on each other. I agree, then, with Robert Imre's point that 'it is not necessarily the case that philosophy [...] needs to be "practical" in showing [social workers] where public policy, or public discourse, or even a guide to individual life, is meant to turn' (Imre 2010: 254). As Law and Urry once commented, to 'change our understanding *is* to change the world, in small and sometimes major ways' (2004: 391).

Thirdly, from the off, we need to be cautious about seeing philosophy in social work as simply a form of *ethics* – even if this is the most obvious area where the two disciplines speak to one another (and, indeed, why many interactions between the two take place within an ethical dialogue – see, for example, Plant (1970); Alexandra and Miller (2009)). We should likewise be wary of positioning philosophy within the same explanatory place of 'social theory' within social work, even if it can and does apply to that area. Our wariness is in part because the tendency for theory in social work to be considered as a purely functional exercise – that is, to 'make sense' of things in order to help things work, without challenging what making sense might mean, who outcomes work for, etc. – is problematic. This is because the very activity involves some kind of philosophical current; and hence why the likes of Amy Rossiter have argued that an understanding of the *ontology* of social work needs to take precedence over and above its ethics (Rossiter 2011). To subsume theory into practice is, ironically, to already posit a specific *metaphysics* of social work: that is, a structuring order that precedes our experience of the world. Hence, when a social work theorist argues that 'all this debate is fine, but is it *useful* for practice?', the philosophical response would typically be: 'that's fine. But on what conditions are we *defining* "useful"?' And while that kind of question can obviously be quite irritating if asked in the wrong context, or asked as an overly-vague rhetorical question, there are clearly contexts within social work where it is entirely appropriate to be asking them, and to be demanding articulate answers.

Fourthly, in turn, we need to resist the idea that social work speaks back to philosophy because of some privileged empirical experiences that can only be understood from a practitioner's perspective. This attitude – what we might call a celebration of immanence – is at best facile. Instead, I would argue that social work intersects with philosophical concerns because of the different *sites of tension* that it occupies (Parton 1994; Price and Simpson 2007). The International Federation of

Social Workers (IFSW), for example, lists four key tensions embedded within the idea of social work itself, all of which point to philosophical problems:[1]

1. Social workers are often asked to act from within the middle of conflicting interests, interests which they may well be equally invested and 'loyal' to. The dignity of an individual, the welfare of a child, the wellbeing of a community and the integrity of the profession may all compete for primacy in the outcome of an intervention. These have continuously raised questions for social work and philosophy alike as to the basis on which we frame and understand concepts such as the self, the community, individual dignity and so on.
2. There often exists a conflict between the duty of social workers to 'protect the interests of the people with whom they work,' and broader social and political demands for 'efficiency and utility'. Both demands are grounded on important philosophical arguments regarding the rationalisation of action, and what constitutes our interests and relations in a globalised world. This requires articulating the bonds between people – culturally, ethically, politically, or communicatively – beyond the domain of behavioural or psychosocial descriptions.
3. Social workers function as both 'helpers and controllers'. But the distinction between 'helping' and 'controlling' is far from obvious. Making a best interest assessment on a service user with learning difficulties may well be helpful, even if it appears to be an act of control; conversely, strategies for empowerment can easily risk stereotyping or tokenism, and thus over-determining service user identity. The old adage that social workers must choose between being 'agents of the state' or 'agents of change' is, thankfully, losing currency; the dichotomy is false, as both simply beg the question as to what kind/s of power a social worker could be said to have. How, for example, do the machinations of their practice – the material culture of social work, its documentation practices and its textuality – shape the world they practice within? To what extent are the means by which they assess or diagnose a situation – that is, their interpretative practices – constituted within competing senses or requirements of what 'meaning' and 'understanding' are?
4. At every level, social workers face the problems created by the limitations on their resources. In this sense, they face the same tensions of all front-line services working with those who are in some sense excluded or marginalised from 'normal' society. The problem of resources is not *simply* one of economics, however: it is also a question of how to balance the ideal with the possible, and the normative (what should happen) from the descriptive (what is happening).

Such tensions derive from both the conflicts within work on the 'ground level' itself (Galambos 2009), and the wider identity and role of social work within welfare provision, and within the formation of 'the social' itself (O'Brien 2004). The nature of these tensions, often situated as ambiguous and contested 'interfaces' between individual and social, marginalised and mainstream (Smith 2010), themselves challenge Kant's distinction between 'private' and 'public' reasoning. As Rossiter once reflected, the place of social work in late capitalist societies is one of doubt and insecurity, framed in a discourse of hope and innocence. From such a place, public and private roles, norms and actions are often blurred in moments of decision, and 'there is no theory that can shield us from the complexity of [for example] the gesture of a white middle class woman giving an alcoholic Native homeless man a bowl of soup' (Rossiter 2001). Hartman argues that it is the 'attention to person and situation and our refusal to retreat from mounting social problems by redefining them as personal defects, that creates the special character of social work'; but, significantly, 'such a position creates both dilemmas and opportunities' (1989: 388). If, as McLaughlin (2012: 11–12) suggests, there is a distinction between a social work researcher and a non-social work researcher, then it is *this* – rather than any privileged access to deprivation and marginalisation – that constitutes the 'difference that is different' which Gray and Webb claim differentiates social work 'from other ways of thinking, such as those found in psychology, sociology, history or philosophy' (2013: 2). It is this that makes the intersection of social work and philosophy so interesting and productive for both perspectives.

Philosophy and interpretation: the strategy of the book

It should be clear, then, that social work and philosophy do intersect in their interests and concerns, and both have something to say to each other. At the same time, it should equally be clear that this book is not attempting to provide immediate 'fix it' solutions in either field, or any kind of mapping exercises *from* philosophical theory *to* social work practice (as we could perhaps say that Blaug (1995) does with his reading of Habermas, or Thompson (1992) with Sartre). It should go without saying that this is not a book about how philosophy, in all of its wisdom, can bestow hitherto unreachable knowledge to the world of social work; Jacques Rancière has rightly warned against the 'pious vision in which philosophy comes to the rescue of the practitioner, […] explaining the reason for his quandary by shedding light on the principle of his practice' (Rancière 1999: ix). 'Philosophy,' he quips, 'does not come to anyone's rescue and no one asks it to'. Neither, of course, is it a book where social workers firmly put philosophers in their place, by showing them what the 'real world' looks like. This is not a book about the philosophy *of* social work, nor does not intend to simply unpack the philosophical basis of the theories, models and approaches specific to social work as a discipline.

For this reason, early on in the project I took the decision not to include any 'case studies', as are conventionally found in social work literature. The result would only be to slot philosophy into an already-crowded space of psychosocial theories that offer more direct 'solutions' to social work contexts (not to mention some of the risks and problems associated with the use of 'invented examples' for both fields; see Grimwood and Miller, 2015). The project is in fact far more modest than its title may suggest: it seeks to lay out some areas of intersection where the two disciplines may mutually inform one another. My strategy is thus – to somewhat grossly paraphrase The Invisible Committee – not one of contamination, but of *resonance*. It effectively involves reading perspectives from philosophy and from social work research side by side, and suggesting ways in which the two resonate with each other: sometimes in harmony, sometimes more jarringly.

On this note, it is worth emphasising that the book will not benefit from being read in isolation, and will likely appear abstract if done so. Philosophy as a practice works far better through questioning and critiquing than through endless lists of references and examples. For this reason, I have pointed to specific areas where these debates may resonate in particular, but I have tried not to re-tread certain sociological or psychological areas that are already well covered in social work literature. Instead, I have included several points throughout each chapter where the reader is asked to reflect on their own practice, in order to help clarify the kind of intersection being explored. My hope is that these strike a healthy balance between reflection and analysis, without over-prescribing these.

One of the fundamental contentions of this book is that social work is not simply a practical activity, but a series of interrelated perspectives on the micro, meso and macro relationships that make up culture, politics and society. It is rooted in interpretative tasks, and this informs the definition of philosophy that I use, which echoes that of Gianni Vattimo:

> Defined as the ontology of actuality, philosophy is practiced as an interpretation of the epoch, a giving-form to widely felt sentiments about the meaning of being alive in a certain society and in a certain historical world. [...] The difference, though, lies in the 'interpretation': philosophy is not the expression of the age, it is interpretation, and although it does strive to be persuasive, it also acknowledges its own contingency, liberty, perilousness. (Vattimo 2004: 88)

As such, I make no claim to offering some kind of final word or holistic overview of either philosophy or social work. This is an unapologetically partial series of essays, reflecting the interpretative and contingent nature of the discipline. Each of the topics examined in these essays commands entire libraries of literature within both disciplines, and in filling in some gaps we will always be opening more. The fact that social work is, fundamentally, a *relational* practice means that any appeal to a 'God's eye view', universal survey or impartial view of what the world is 'really like', detached from any meaningful location or perspective, is unhelpful in practical terms. Likewise, the unifying theme of philosophical and cultural hermeneutics is the interpretative relationships between people, concepts, and the material world around them; it focuses on how the meaning of our actions is articulated within these relationships, and what the cultural, political and social significance of them is. Graham Ward summarises this approach neatly:

> Ontological and epistemological categories are understood to emerge from and issue into various forms of action, wedding practical wisdom (*phronesis*) with the learned skill of handling language (*techne*) and habits of everyday

life (*praxis*). The activity of interpretation is conducted alongside and with respect to other people and the many cultural forms that are the products of the interaction between people (institutions, tools, art-forms). [...] Cultural hermeneutics is concerned with the concrete reality of others. (Ward 2005: 65)

This 'concrete reality' is important for the hermeneutic approach. Recognising the importance of interpretation to the meanings that surround and define us does not lead to some kind of linguistic idealism – we cannot simply interpret out of thin air. Rather, concrete reality is always mediated: by the language we speak, the cultural images and metaphors that pervade it, the social structures within it, and so on. The limits of this mediation not only shape the way we think, but also become a matter of thought itself (Taylor 1985). As a brief example, consider how difficult it is to challenge the kind of principle of social work education that Cain asserts: '[s]ocial work education is about more than just teaching new information and skills; it is also about encouraging students to question their assumptions and values and the structure of the world around them' (1996: 65). But the very fact that few *would* challenge this – as Cain's argument which then unfolds, regarding the implicit heterosexism of social work education, makes clear – means that further questions also need to be asked: *from where* would a student do this? Is it possible to question assumptions without resting on further assumptions? At what point do we stop? At what point *can* we stop questioning? Are there certain modes of thought which we cannot help but use when we think about certain areas of practice – regardless of whether these are 'good' or not? Without asking such questions, 'critical thinking' can become something of an over-determined and artificially linear path of therapeutic self-discovery – 'I used to *think* this, but now I *know* that!' – rather than an ongoing interpretative project.

But how practical *is it*?

If philosophy is the practice of interpreting the meaning of human ideas and actions in order to facilitate both understanding and transformation, then in this sense, professionals working in social care, community work and social work all engage with philosophical ideas on a day-to-day level, in what Lena Dominelli has characterised as the 'change orientation' within social work knowledge (2005: 230). This interpretative aspect underlies the approach of this book precisely because philosophy and social work share an essential relation whereby they are both, fundamentally, about thinking and acting both *within* and *beyond* culture. *Within* culture, because both are formed substantively by responding to the needs, calls and pressures of a contemporary socio-cultural context. They are shaped around a certain functional requirement. But both social work and philosophy are also *beyond* culture, to the extent that the contours of their practice are concerned with change and transformation. Responses to the present are made meaningful only through a broader focus on the future. This is perhaps more readily seen in the radical and critical social work theorists, far more than the procession of 'models' and diagrammatic explanations of 'how things are' that can tend to dominate social work education. But even the most pragmatic and functionalist approaches carry implicit aspirations towards a certain type of society, and a certain direction it should take.

The danger felt by some, of course, may be that there is such a thing as too much questioning, or too much reflection, and that this will inevitably come at the expense of something else. In this case, we must be careful to delineate between the neoliberal framing of higher education, which demands subject disciplines show their 'market value' and 'economic impact' in immediate and quantifiable terms, and the more political voices of social work theory that look for theory to make a recognisably political *difference* to the context of practice. The first sense of 'being useful' is problematic for both social work and philosophy. The second sense is part of a wider dialogue over the role of theory and socio-cultural transformation, which I hope this book contributes to, even if it is not a book devoted solely to politics and policy. The 'practical' task of the book, rather, is to consider whether what makes sense – either in theory or practice – actually *does* makes sense, rather than simply reproducing the readymade authority of clichés and platitudes; and it does this by examining what the *conditions* of it making sense are.

Once, it was thought that an understanding on what lay beyond the immediacies of the world of practice was the best bulwark against social workers losing hope: as when MacIver claimed that the 'social worker who has no background of social philosophy is at the mercy of a thousand discouragements' (MacIver, quoted in Marshall 1946: 17). Today, this view of philosophy as therapy may be less popular! But the need to think outside of the inevitability of the present remains just as pressing. And as previously mentioned, such thinking may be best done, not through the contamination of one discipline into the other, but rather through the resonance of arguments and ideas.

Note

1   http://www.iassw-aiets.org/ethics-in-social-work-statement-of-principles (accessed 03/12/2014).

References

Alexandra, A., and Miller, S. (2009). *Ethics in Practice: Moral Theory and the Professions* Melbourne: UNSW Press.
Barber, A. (2010). *Ethics*. Milton Keynes: Open University Press.
Blaug, R. (1995). 'Distortion of the Face to Face: Communicative Reason and Social Work Practice.' *British Journal of Social Work*, 25, 423–39.
Cain, R. (1996). 'Heterosexism and Self Dis-Closure in the Social Work Classroom.' *Journal of Social Work Education*, 32 (1), 65–76.
Coulshed, V., and Orme, J. (2006). *Social Work Practice*. 4th edn. Basingstoke: Palgrave MacMillan.
Dominelli, L. (1996). 'De-Professionalising Social Work: Anti-Oppressive Practices, Competencies and Postmodernism.' *British Journal of Social Work*, 26, 153–75.

—— (2005). 'Social Work Research: Contested Knowledge for Practice.' In Adams, R., Dominelli, L., and Payne, M. (eds.), *Social Work Futures: Crossing Boundaries, Transforming Practice*. Basingstoke: Palgrave MacMillan, pp. 223–36.

Fook, J. (2000). 'Critical Perspectives on Social Work Practice.' In O'Connor, I., Smyth, P., and Warburton, J. (eds.), *Contemporary Perspectives on Social Work and the Human Sciences*. Melbourne: Addison-Wesley Longman, pp. 128–37.

Foucault, M. (1984). 'What is Enlightenment?', C. Porter (trans.). In Rabinow, P. (ed.), *The Foucault Reader*. London: Penguin, pp. 32–50.

Galambos, C. (2009). 'Political Tolerance, Social Work Values, and Social Work Education.' *Journal of Social Work Education*, 45 (3), 343–37.

Garrett, P. (2013). *Social Work and Social Theory*. Bristol: Policy Press.

Gray, M., and Webb, S. (2013). 'Introduction.' In Gray, M., and Webb, S. (eds.), *Social Work Theories and Methods*. London: Sage, pp.1–10.

Grimwood, T., and Miller, P. (2014). 'How To Do Things Without Words.' In Garvey, B. (ed.), *J.L. Austin on Language*. Basingstoke: Palgrave Macmillan.

—— (2015). 'Mountains, Cones and Dilemmas of Context: The Case of "Ordinary Language" in Philosophy and Social Scientific Method.' *Philosophy of the Social Sciences* 45(3), 331–55.

Hartman, A. (1989). 'Still between Client and Community.' *Social Work*, 24 (5), 387–8.

Howe, D. (1987). *An Introduction to Social Work Theory*. Aldershot: Ashgate.

Hugman, R. (2013). 'Rights-based International Social Work Practice.' In Gray, M., and Webb, S. (eds.), *The New Politics of Social Work*. Basingstoke: Palgrave Macmillan, pp.159–73.

Imre, R. (2010). 'Badiou and the Philosophy of Social Work: A Reply to Stephen Webb.' *International Journal of Social Welfare* 19, 253–8.

Jones, C. (1996). 'Anti-Intellectualism and the Peculiarities of British Social Work Education.' In Parton, N. (ed.), *Social Theory, Social Change and Social Work*. London: Routledge, pp. 190–210.

Kant, I. (1996 [1784]). 'An Answer to the Question: "What is Enlightenment?"' in Gregor, M.J. (ed.), *Immanuel Kant: Practical Philosophy*. Cambridge: Cambridge University Press, pp.11–22.

Kant I. (1993 [1787]). *Critique of Pure Reason*, J.M.D. Meiklejohn (trans.). London: J.M. Dent.

Lanham, R. (1991). *A Handlist of Rhetorical Terms*. 2nd edn. London: University of California Press.

Law, J. and Urry, J. (2004). 'Enacting the Social.' *Economy and Society*, 33 (3), 390–410.

Lewis, J. (1995). *The Voluntary Sector, the State and Social Work in Britain: The Charity Organisation Society/Family Welfare Association since 1869*. Aldershot: Edward Elgar.

Marshall, T. (1946). 'Training for Social Work', in Nuffield College (ed.), *Training for Social Work*. Oxford: Oxford University Press.

McLaughlin, H. (2012). *Understanding Social Work Research*. 2nd edition. London: Sage.

Mullaly, B. (1997). *Structural Social Work: Ideology, Theory and Practice*. 2nd edn. Oxford: Oxford University Press.

Niźnik, J. (2006). *The Arbitrariness of Philosophy*. Aurora, CO: The Davies Group Publishers.

O'Brien, M. (2004). 'What is Social about Social Work?' *Social Work and Social Sciences Review*, 11 (2), 5–19.

Parton, N. (1994) 'Problematics of Government', (Post) Modernity and Social Work.' *British Journal of Social Work*, 24 (1), 9–32.

Pierson, J. (2011). *Understanding Social Work: History and Context*. Maidenhead: Open University Press.

Plant, R. (1970). *Social and Moral Theory in Casework*. London: Routledge and Kegan Paul.

Price, V. and Simpson, G. (2007). *Transforming Society? Social Work and Sociology*. Bristol: Policy Press.

Rancière, J. (1999). *Dis-agreement: Politics and Philosophy*, J. Rose (trans.). Minneapolis, MN: University of Minnesota Press.

Rossiter, A. (2001). 'Innocence Lost and Suspicion Found: Do we Educate for or Against Social Work?' *Critical Social Work*, 2, (1). Available at http://www1.uwindsor.ca/criticalsocialwork/innocence-lost-and-suspicion-found-do-we-educate-for-or-against-social-work

Rossiter, A. (2011). 'Unsettled Social Work: The Challenge of Levinas's Ethics.' *British Journal of Social Work*, 41, 980–95.

Schön, D. (1987). *Educating the Reflective Practitioner: Toward a New Design for Teaching and Learning in the Professions*. Oxford: Wiley Blackwell.

Simon, B. (1994). *The Empowerment Tradition in American Social Work: A History*. New York: Columbia University Press.

Smith, R. (2010). 'Social Work, Risk, Power.' *Sociological Research Online*, 15, (1). Available at *http://www.socresonline.org.uk/15/1/4.html*

Taylor, C. (1985). *Philosophy and the Human Sciences*. Cambridge: Cambridge University Press.

Thompson, N. (1992). *Existentialism and Social Work*. Aldershot: Avebury.

Thompson, N. (2010). *Theorising Social Work Practice*. Basingstoke: Palgrave Macmillan.

Vattimo, G. (2004). *Nihilism and Emancipation: Ethics, Politics and Law*. New York: Columbia University Press.

Vattimo, G. and Zabala, S. (2011). *Hermeneutic Communism: From Heidegger to Marx*. New York: Columbia University Press.

Ward, G. (2005). *Cultural Transformation and Religious Practice*. Cambridge: Cambridge University Press.

1
INTERPRETATION
Social work and hermeneutics

Meaning, understanding, and interpretation

Speaking meaningfully about meaning, or trying to understand understanding, is a tricky thing to do. As one review of the different ways in which meaning has been discussed in social work discourse illustrates (see Furman et al. 2014), there is a tendency to jump to the 'big' question of what meaning is: what gives *my life* meaning? What is the meaning of social work *as a profession*? But these questions already assume we know what 'meaning' means in itself. Likewise, research in psychology can inform us of the cognitive processes that lead to 'understanding'; but only under an assumed sense of what 'understanding' is. The more fundamental question is a *hermeneutic* one: how do we arrive at these parameters of 'meaningfulness' in the first place? What are the conditions for us to understand meaning at all? These questions are core to the philosophy of interpretation.

If these appear as abstract questions, it is worth considering how interpretation underlies some of the most basic of tensions within practical contexts. For example, in 2014, Peter Fahy, the chief constable of the Greater Manchester police force, called for the police to have the right to access the medical records of those vulnerable people they worked with. Fahy argued that this 'would give us a deeper understanding of those we are expected to help and their problems'.[1] Access to information – medical history of individuals, the conditions they had, their next of kin – would help to improve the service that the police offered. There are several points of contention within this claim, many of which Fahy was clearly hoping to open a discussion on: the changing role of the police in the community, the way that other professions such as social workers approached confidentiality, and so on. But while all of these are worth discussion, there is a more fundamental problem with his call, which centres on the relationship between 'information', 'understanding' and 'meaning'. As mental health professionals were quick to point out in response to Fahy, simply possessing the information that an individual has a condition, or has a history of violence, or has been resident in care, does not equate to understanding what these terms *mean*. It is no use somebody knowing that an individual has been diagnosed with schizophrenia, if they hold only negative perceptions of what that entails. It is no use somebody knowing that an individual has been in care, if this information then becomes some kind of overriding faux-scientific causal explanation for every action they perform. The word 'stigma', it is worth remembering, comes from the Greek word for 'mark' or 'sign'. The kind of information that Fahy asked for was, effectively, just that: literal signs or marks by which to identify individual bodies. What was lacking in the call for access to service user records was a sense of how meaning emerges, not from such signs and marks *in themselves*, but from both the references and resonances they lead us to, and from the interpretation of them by their readers.

Of course, the discourses of health care, social care, policing and so on all recognise that words, signs and marks change their meaning over time. The changing categorisation of mental health conditions, shifts in the identification of social classes, and the way that racial and gendered slang can move from derogatory to self-identifying (or vice versa), are all clear examples of this. Until 1973, homosexuality was referred to as a psychiatric disorder by the American Psychiatric Association; it now refers to a sexual orientation. Changes to the available information about something will affect its meaning, which is also why some words have different meanings depending on their technical context: the word 'assessment', for example, carries a different implication for a social worker than for an educator. Recognising the role of context can, however, still leave this relationship between meaning and information as taken somewhat for granted. It involves something of a 'flat' sense of what meaning *is*: there is a sense that meaning is rooted in a straightforward relationship between a recognised sign, word or symbol, and a corresponding term.

But there are two fundamental problems with this flat sense of meaning that presumes there is a simple correspondence between sign and reference. How do we recognise such a correspondence in the first place, and how is the correspondence formed? As we never simply 'encounter' a sign, or word, or symbol in isolation, but rather always within the flows of our socio-cultural practices, then meaning is at least in part tied to the social world we inhabit. As Ian Burkitt notes (2008: 59), any participation within shared meanings – such as following ethical guidelines, claiming a shared identity such as 'social worker', or even expressing recognisable emotions to an interlocutor, such as 'sympathy' or 'confidence' – all involve a *performance* of whatever agreed attributes of that meaning are recognisable. As such, meaning always depends upon interpretation of some kind.

The second, and related, problem is that, if we focus exclusively on the idea that meaning is an external process of sign referring to signifier, we overlook our own role in *constructing* sense out of the world around us, and the interaction between our own interpretations and the production of culture and society around us. In other words, interpretation is an *active* part of the creation of meaning. Whether at the micro level of interpersonal interaction, the broader levels of multi-agency working and linking available resources to client need, or at the macro level of socio-political critique, social work is embedded within multiple sites of continuous and active interpretation. Indeed, it could be argued that from the earliest days of social work, trappings of casework such as the Charity Organisation Society's 'flow charts' for decision making (Humphreys 1995: 113), or their methods for 'taking down the case' (Lymbery 2005: 37), were designed to direct the interpretative nature of the social worker's inquiries into a reasonably systematic order. But of course, such methods, and their analogous forebears (assessment tools, eligibility criteria, etc.) would not *remove* interpretation. Not only would the details of the 'case' often be far from self-evident, and therefore requiring interpretation on the part of the worker, but also the line of questioning employed – as is the case for any assessment tool – is geared around the illumination of a particular perspective, predicated on an underlying sense of how problems should be ordered, what problems take priority, and how they might be approached. As then, so today: even assessments, interventions and monitoring all still require sometimes complex interpretation in order to be put into practice (White and Stancombe 2002).

It is for such reasons that Gray and Webb argue that, contrary to appearances, social work is not simply the carrying out of 'common sense' responses to problems, but rather an activity which is 'about "*making* sense" of human reality' (2013: 2, my emphasis). Relating the immanence of practice to the wider contexts that both shape and give meaning to the everyday, and vice versa, all involves active interpretation. Meaning is never simply 'given': as they note, we 'speak a language we did not create, we use technology we did not invent and we claim rights we did not establish and so on. Even feelings that appear completely spontaneous, such as the anger expressed at certain types of crime, are, in reality, the product of a social context' (2013: 2). It is clear, then, that interpretation is central to not only the formation of the 'meanings' which underlie practice (the concepts, identities, classes and typologies that give social work its language), but also to the activity of social work at all its different levels; and that 'this adds up to what we might call the hermeneutic worker – the worker acting within a reflexive–interpretive process of self and other' (McBeath and Webb 2002: 1016). But what is perhaps less clear is what, exactly, *constitutes* interpretation in this sense.

Defining interpretation: some questions

As well as being an act of relating everyday instances to the wider social contexts which give meaning to actions, feelings and words, Gray and Webb also offer this by way of a more specific definition:

> Interpretation in social work requires the recovery of meaning or intention of clients' actions. As a client may describe her action retrospectively in ways which she did not, or could not describe before it was completed, interpretation has a privileged position in social work. (Gray and Webb 2013: 3)

Social workers, therefore, utilise a 'specialised' form of interpretation, which involves drawing on specific communication skills and broader knowledge. Interpretation becomes crucial to this specialised practice – what Gray and Webb describe as the 'difference that makes a difference' (2013: 2) between the phronetic character of social work knowledge and the theories they draw this from. If we are to take seriously this 'privileged position', though, we might also note how this brief passage raises several immediate questions:

1. Can we ever recover a meaning or intention *fully*?
2. If it is true that 'we speak a language that we didn't create' (as Gray and Webb suggested earlier), can we ever *actually* mean what we say?
3. Are we recovering meaning, or are we instead *translating* one meaning into a different meaning recognised by practice – that is, into the appropriate terminology of the service, or the language of assessment, or the vocabulary which is understood by management and stakeholders? Is this done in the sense that Jan Fook suggests 'workers might see part of their role as transforming bureaucratic culture by *valuing and translating* between different discourses' (2002: 147–8, my emphasis)?
4. Is such a language of practice based on the belief that there are universal conditions of experience that can legitimise such translation? Are we translating for the sake of matching client action to our models? If so, what are these conditions and where did we find them? Or are we (as Fook suggests) problematising categorisation itself, by introducing new and distinct forms of description? If so, then how do we link each of our interpretations in such a way that we arrive at a single occupation of 'social work'?
5. Indeed, if we speak a language that we didn't create, how reliable is the 'we' that such a language provides us to speak with? To what extent does the language we use define the 'we' who speak, and how does this representation of 'us' invoke both political and cultural implications? This question is raised in work such as Gai Harrison's, which has argued that far greater recognition needs to be given to how 'language politics' affects personal and professional identity in social work, especially in terms of recognising how inequitable relations are maintained through 'linguistic othering' (Harrison 2009).
6. Is the space for interpretation limited to interactions with clients and the documentation of that interaction, or are there interpretative acts going on at every level – including the sense of whether there is such a thing as a clear definition of what social work is? Given the 'difference that makes a difference' which Gray and Webb also note is key to social work knowledge, to what extent is the interpretative basis of social work fundamental to its responsively dynamic identity?

Thinking through the possible responses to these questions will help to unpack the hermeneutic commitments within the claim that social work is about interpreting and making sense of human reality. It is in this sense that Nancy Moules terms

> **Thinking through Practice**
>
> Apply the questions above to reflections on your own cases. How would you answer them all? Do any strike you as more *significant* to your own practice than others? Why?

practitioners 'brokers of understanding': 'situated in the middle of ongoing and multifarious negotiations of mutual and self-understanding, [...] making sense of particulars, putting them in context, assigning relevance and meaning, and acting on the implications of that meaning' (Moules *et al.* 2011: 2). Interpretation underlies this all. The use of any formal mechanism to ascertain the 'real' meaning of what's going on – an assessment tool, or a decision-making heuristic, for example – certainly does not remove interpretation from the scene. Rather, it simply prioritises certain interpretations, and certain meanings, at the expense of others.

Of course, prioritisation *has* to be made. Even if we are aware of a whole range of possible meanings, the contexts of practice will often demand that we commit to one over others. This means that, beyond the general directives that social work practice and education has built itself for discerning what is 'meaningful' (such as 'starting where the client is', empowerment, cultural sensitivity and so on (see Furman *et al.* 2014: 74)),[2] professional practice 'in reality is messy, problems are not well defined', and that 'there exists in most situations a variety of options, each involving trade-offs among competing goals and values' (Lynton 1990: 13).

Before exploring the philosophical responses to this problem, though, I want to consider two of the more common uses of the word 'interpretation', as both may come to mind in reaction to the inherent messiness of practice. First, in recent times, 'interpretation' has often come to be used to infer simple 'opinion'. 'That's your interpretation!' is often used in our day-to-day conversations as a way of ending discussion rather than opening it: it points to an impossibility of agreement, as well as a more general suggestion that the full 'truth' of the matter can't be achieved from one person's viewpoint alone. There are obvious problems with any application of this notion of interpretation to practice. I would term this a 'thin' sense of interpretation, as it would sit on the thin end of a wedge that then thickens out in accordance with the more objective, evidence-based, usually quantitative, and certain our knowledge becomes. Interpretation, in this case, is seen effectively as the opposite of 'truth'. This is, however, simply a misuse of the term. Interpretation is not the same as opinion; it is a far more fundamental part of meaning which prefigures any form of evidence or opinion. Incidentally, this misuse can also arise when the act of interpretation is seen as a 'value-judgement' (see Folgheraiter 2004: 28), whereby values are seen – again, wrongly – as somehow inherently subjective, therefore inferior to 'facts'.

Second, interpretation can be used to mean something like an instrument towards discovering a more certain or secure truth. This is grounded upon the notion – which, as John Heritage remarks, is 'a pervasive and long-standing view' – that language ultimately serves a representative function. 'Within this view,' Heritage continues, 'the meaning of a word is what it references, corresponds with, or stands for in the real world. [...] [This] view of language has remained a tacit assumption for generations of social scientists' (Heritage 1984: 137). As a tacit assumption, it of course carries an immediate obviousness. Signs refer to things which give them meaning. For example, if the social worker is concerned with reconstructing the lost or fragmented sense of the service user's actions and experiences, then the task is to match their words with the reality they are trying to express. Or, perhaps a less 'ethical' example: a social worker visiting a service user's home may find themselves implicitly conducting a kind of forensic inquiry – detecting particular signs (unwashed laundry in a client's house? out-of-date food in their fridge?) will suggest a specific form of living (are they a neglectful parent?) that in turn informs the appropriate action for the practitioner to take.

This correspondence account of meaning sees interpretation as simply an instrument or tool to be picked up, used, and dropped as required. For some, this underlies the entire relationship between theory and practice. Hence, for Barbra Teater, theories exist to 'assist social workers in understanding, explaining or making sense of situations' (Teater 2010: 3). Social workers dealing with a child who has been placed in numerous foster care settings may look to Bowlby's theory of attachment to interpret the child's disruptive behaviour. Those working with clients with an eating disorder may utilise Cognitive Behavioural Therapy as a method for intervention. In each case, 'the key is ensuring that what the social worker utilizes is appropriate for the client and situation, and that the theory or method is working' (Teater 2010: 6). If one doesn't work, then simply move on to the next one. The problem with this response, though, is that it seems to leap from a world of inherent messiness and difficulty into one of apparent tidiness. While, in fairness, Teater makes no claim that assessing the appropriateness of theories is easy, her distinction between theory, method and practice nevertheless tends to already assume clear categories to work with: what ideas we have of how good practice appears, how we know if we have understood a service user, and so on. Likewise, the correspondence account of meaning requires a more detailed theoretical account of how we know that we have discovered the true corresponding meaning, beyond professional intuition. Such an instrumental account therefore moves too quickly over the issue of exactly how interpretation is conceptualised, justified and utilised.

In short, this kind of subordination of interpretation to a simple functional task is unhelpful, once it is recognised that, as Adams *et al.* argue, 'paradoxes and dilemmas are embedded within practice' (2009: 333). While in some cases it is entirely possible to, like the scientist testing for variables, simply move from one approach to the next until something 'works', in most cases *meaning itself conflicts*. The question of what is the most 'appropriate' theory or method to use cannot be answered from a neutral space in this way: hence why, for Adams *et al.*, 'critical practice' must replace reflective practice. Critical practice 'is *difficult* [...] because it involves accepting both constraints and freedom, in the context of everyday realities' (2009: 310, my emphasis). This is why Moules argues that the task of the practitioner is not one of *achieving* understanding, but rather brokering it: practice is 'an interpretive practice that occurs in a shifting in-between, in the middle of relationships, contexts, and particularities' (Moules *et al.* 2011: 2).

The hermeneutics of restoration: interpreting 'objectively'

So to the question: what *is* interpretation, and what is its relationship to both 'meaning' and 'understanding'? The philosophical debates begin from a dissatisfaction with the restrictive and domineering strategies of naïve realism – the idea that 'what you see is what you get' – and explore the different ways in which interpretation takes place, what its task is, what its content is, and how meaning is created through it.

Initially, hermeneutics concerned itself with the interpretation of texts; specifically in terms of religious texts, and later the relationship between language and cultural context. From the eighteenth century onwards, an interest in the relationship between signs, symbols and context emerged in the philosophy of both linguistics and history. Friedrich Schleiermacher, though, was the first to develop a 'universal' account of hermeneutics, which did not apply to one particular source (a certain kind of text, a particular language) but to meaning in general. From this point, hermeneutics developed from a theory of reading to a broader theory of understanding. In the early twentieth century Martin Heidegger suggested that a fundamental hermeneutics underlay not only our general understanding of anything, but also our very existence as human beings. Under the influence of these arguments (though not, thankfully, Heidegger's politics), hermeneutics grew outwards into a wide range of academic areas, shaping the 'interpretative paradigm' underlying qualitative research (see McLaughlin 2012).

> **Thinking through Practice**
>
> In his book *Street-Level Bureaucrats: The Dilemmas of Individuals in Public Service*, Michael Lipsky (1980) argued that the nature of social workers' jobs in large-scale organisations meant they were afforded significant discretion to interpret how policy could or should be applied to the service users on the 'street level'. Since then, many social workers have argued that such 'discretion' has been increasingly removed by excessive strictures of managerialism (see Ferguson and Woodward 2009).
>
> How do you see the relationship between discretion and interpretation within your work? To what extent might working contexts affect the availability of approaches to understanding what 'interpretation' is?

Paul Ricoeur has suggested that hermeneutics as a whole is governed by a 'double motivation', which he characterises as the willingness to *listen*, and the willingness to *suspect* (1970: 27). On the one hand, the differences between ourselves and the thing we are interpreting – the event, speech, text, persons and so on – need to be recognised and heard. Otherwise, we are not actually interpreting, but presuming. This approach seems to be at work in Gray and Webb's definition of interpretation, as well as those approaches focused on the voice of service users as 'experts by experience' in research or practice (Preston-Shoot 2007; Scourfield 2010). On the other hand, the very need for hermeneutical inquiry in itself suggests that such listening is open to *misinterpretation*. As we began this chapter by noting, meaning is rarely transparent, and does not always equate with understanding. The language we use is susceptible to influence, power, and ideologies that may be contrary to the words actually spoken. Thus, in the first case 'hermeneutics is understood as the manifestation and restoration of a meaning addressed to me in the manner of a message'; in the second, 'it is understood as a demystification, as a reduction of illusion' (Ricoeur 1970: 26).[3]

Discerning whether or not we have understood a text, speech or event was, for the early theorists, the central task of hermeneutics. Understanding the meaning of a text or event for the likes of Schleiermacher involved an essentially psychological approach. This *restorative* task was to rid interpretation of any prejudice that may have sullied the meaning of the original, and reconstruct the psychological conditions through which the text was written, the words were spoken, or the event was produced. Of course, if a student mis-hears what their practice educator says to them, they can simply ask them to repeat themselves. It becomes more complicated, however, when the distance – whether temporal, spatial, emotional, cultural, perceived or real – is more significant. We have already seen a pertinent example in Gray and Webb's definition: that is, if 'a client may describe her action retrospectively in ways which she did not, or could not describe before it was completed' (2013: 2). Here, a more rigorous approach to discerning whether we have, in fact, 'understood' what we are interpreting is necessary.

More recent theorists such as John Searle or E.D. Hirsch Jr developed this notion of restoration into an 'objectivist' hermeneutics. Interpretation, in this sense, is primarily concerned with finding the correct perspective to see the thing being interpreted *as it is in itself* – that is, as an object. While words may have a whole range of possible meanings, the 'primary' meaning of a communicative act is its 'intentionality' (Searle 1979). While there may be 'secondary' meanings produced by dialogue (e.g. for example, the need for a shared language between service user and professional may involve words that go beyond, or do not go far enough, in describing the service user's experiences), or by the medium of expression (e.g., the documentation of what is said in an initial assessment report will produce a meaning *shaped* by the service provision; a conversation on a telephone allows certain meanings to be clearer or more obscure compared to a face-to-face encounter), neither of these are the same as what the speaker *means*. Instead, the speaker employs the secondary aspect to express the primary meaning: we, as listeners, reverse this process by using the medium of expression in order to uncover the meaning which the speaker intends us to hear. In other words, the task of hermeneutics is to restore the original meaning behind the words, actions and expressions a person uses. On this reading, the answer to our list of questions above is straightforward enough: the answer to question (1) is 'yes': we can understand someone's meaning fully and objectively, because language is subordinate to meaning. Therefore, the answer to question (2) is also 'yes': we can mean what we say, if the language we use serves our purpose well enough. Questions (3) to (7) then effectively become redundant, as the hermeneutics of restoration gives a clear sense of how we interpret, and where meaning resides.

Some problems with objectivity

What if there is ambiguity between expression and intention, though? Within the language of social work, particular words – pertaining to relationships, attachments, personal worth, dignity and so on – are notoriously multi-layered; and hence Fook's argument, which we mentioned earlier, that social work is an act of translation across the different discourses of service user experience, advocacy, activism, bureaucracy and so on. How, then, can we 'know' what people mean? Hirsch (1967) argues that in cases of ambiguity there is rarely a case where *probability* cannot inform us of the most likely correct meaning. Any assessment of a communication's meaning – and any ambiguity that this might raise – is always grounded on the original intention of the communicator. Any subsequent meanings that may arise from a service user's account are, on this argument, incidental to what the social worker should be interested in. This denotes a difference between 'meaning', which is determined purely by the author (in the case of Gray and Webb's example, the service user) and 'significance', which is the meaning that a listener may glean (in this case, the social worker's situating of the service user's account in the broader context of their case history, the available services, the relevant theories underpinning their practice, etc.). For Hirsch, 'significance' is not what grounds the *validity* of our interpretations; likewise, Searle argues emphatically that 'sentences and words have only the meanings that they have' (1993: 84). For example, knowing that there is a shortage of foster carers does not determine what a parent means when they talk of the problems they have in looking after their child.

But this in turn raises a problem which Gray and Webb first alerted us to when they noted that we 'speak a language which we did not create'. If language is shared in this way, does this not affect the idea that the author is the *sole* determiner of meaning? It would seem that both Searle and Hirsch tend to assume a certain 'fixedness' between object (the person or thing being interpreted) and subject (the person interpreting). Without this, they both argue, there can be no way of knowing if you have really understood something. However, this relatively stable view put forward by Searle and Hirsch – which appears as a linear act of intention, to meaning, to expression, to listening, to restored intention – is rendered problematic when applied to the daily practice of social work.

Fabio Folgheraiter's work on relational social work (2004) provides examples of cases where an individual's status as a service user arises from core *intersubjective* problems rather than linear relationships. Folgheraiter argues that approaching cases through a clear subject/object lens leads to recommendations of linear intervention being seen as 'common sensical'. His example is a case of a fifteen-year-old in care who is being disruptive in school. The linear response sees the child as the problem (the object), and the intervention as removing him from the school, having him assessed by a psychiatric specialist, and getting the misbehaviour 'fixed'. Folgheraiter's relational approach, meanwhile, suggests that in this case the problem itself is social (regarding the relationships within the classroom, between teacher and students, as well as the host of relations that have brought the fifteen-year-old to this point in his life). 'For fully thirteen years a set of natural relationships have worked day and night to turn [him] into what he is', Folgheraiter reflects. 'How many years of our artificial relationships will it take to change him?' (2004: 229). His point is that how we align a subject and an object is inherently dependent upon the relations within a situation. Being aware of how the object of our interpretation appears to us *as* an object is thus important not simply at the level of intervention, but at the initial level of establishing what is actually going on in and around the case presented to the social worker: who is at stake, and how their sense of identity within the case is established through their relationships with the environment around them. This is to ask, as David Couzens Hoy does, 'what happens when the object of interpretation disappears, when it fractures and splinters so that we begin to suspect that our own eyes are multifarious?' (1982: 46). The 'service user voice' can often be complex and multi-layered, not just because of their past histories, but because these are, at least in part, conditioned by their current relationships. In this sense, cases may not always be something which are objectively and indifferently 'there', stood before the social worker. Indeed, for Folgheraiter, the challenge for the social worker in this particular example is to effectively challenge the conception that the fifteen-year-old is an isolated object of interpretation, and demonstrate the fragmented and multi-layered formation of the problem at hand.

The hermeneutics of trust: Hans-Georg Gadamer

The work of Hans-Georg Gadamer speaks to these problems. Gadamer rejects the starting principles that govern the hermeneutics of restoration. We will never be able to know someone's intention better than they did, because intention cannot be separated from the effects of the words we use; meanings can never be 'fixed' by a person, as meanings are part of an ongoing effective history. As such, we never simply arrive at an object of interpretation – be it a text, person, painting, etc. – from nowhere, but are bound to particular traditions of understanding. Our interpretations are always *situated* within what Gadamer terms an 'effective-historical consciousness.' Gadamer terms this situated-ness a 'horizon' for understanding: our 'range of vision that includes everything that can be seen from a particular vantage point' (Gadamer 2004: 301). This fluctuating frame of reference is shaped and changed by the limits of our historical situation and knowledge, and the ways in which such knowledge is significant to us: hence, 'a person who has an horizon knows the relative significance of everything within this horizon, whether it is near or far, great or small. Similarly, working out the hermeneutical situation means acquiring the right horizon of inquiry for the questions evoked by the encounter with tradition' (Gadamer 2004: 301–2). For Gadamer, our *entire* thinking is always a process of interconnected interpretations, over and above mere explanation.

At first sight, this may seem perfectly obvious. Even Schleiermacher recognised that 'every utterance presupposes a given language' and 'every utterance depends upon previous thinking' (1998: 8). But Gadamer is going further than this. We do not simply recover meaning in order to explain it, but rather meaning in turn has an effect on us, and the world around it. His concept of understanding is not as an 'object' that can be arrived at and rested upon, but rather something which recognises the life and movement of the thing being understood. The dialogue between social worker and service user is not a route *to* understanding, but is instead what understanding *is*: a fusion of different horizons.

At the heart of Gadamer's hermeneutics is a distrust of the fixed identities and separation of subject (interpreter) and object (interpreted) that previous theories relied upon. Challenging the idea that prejudices are only negative distortions of a reality outside of us, Gadamer suggests that our horizon provides us with a set of prejudices which enable us to understand the object of interpretation. This notion of prejudice is not meant in the pejorative sense of blind dogmatism, but rather the predispositions by which we recognise something as meaningful. This is not just based on our past experiences: for example, the early education that allows us to recognise certain shapes as letters, groups of letters as words and groups of words as a 'language'; or the later education that provides definitions of law, process and policy within social work training. Our horizons are not simply operational knowledge of the world, but also our expectations, projections and hopes of the world. Prejudice is not an obstacle to understanding; it is, rather, a condition of understanding itself. In other words, to 'understand' is to understand oneself in the subject matter of what is being interpreted (Gadamer 2004: 294). We are always *within* the act of interpreting the world; we can never step outside to a point where there is no interpretation going on. Precisely because of this, we are able to adapt and develop our prejudices, and widen our horizon of understanding.

The important point, for Gadamer, is that while we can only ever understand the world from our lived perspective – our horizon – the act of understanding itself requires an encounter with a different viewpoint or horizon. In this way, interpretation rests within a person, text or event's 'strangeness and familiarity to us, between being a historically intended, distanced object and belonging to a tradition. *The true locus of hermeneutics is this in-between*' (Gadamer 2004: 295, emphasis in original). Understanding is a dialogue, or, in Gadamer's celebrated phrase, a *fusion of horizons*: a joining together of the different horizons of interpreter and interpreted. Thus, in the interaction between social worker and service user – an initial assessment visit, for example – both parties engage with each other as part of an ongoing, lived and temporal perspective. In such an interaction, it is not simply a case of creating meaning through a shared purpose or agenda between the pre-agreed positions of social worker and service user (see Woodcock Ross 2011). Rather, it is recognising that meaning emerges as meaningful in the opening of our own horizon to the possibility of a different perspective; which, in turn, implies that our own horizon is always incomplete. Interpretation is not the recovery of something that is lost, in this sense, and does not, therefore, require an objective 'truth' or singular 'meaning'.

This limits the claim that any interpretation can make to 'absolute' knowledge; but in doing so it makes interpretation far more fundamental to practice than the restorative model. As Amy Rossiter has argued, there is no such thing as 'innocent' knowledge within social work (see also Jardine 2012: 8). 'As much as I'd like to have a practice of freedom that is pure and free from doubt,' she argues, 'there is no such ahistorical, decontextualized space. We are always acting in and through a history in which the contradictions of history are lived out in our practices, and no person – even ones who do it perfectly can be extracted from history' (Rossiter 2001). But rather than dissolve this lack of innocence into moral and epistemic relativism, or superimpose a new 'innocence' that simply ignores or obscures the lived traditions of social work, Gadamer argues that both morality and epistemology develop from out of our interpretative standpoint. Hermeneutics is an *ontological* task, not a methodological one. In this sense, understanding can only ever be interpretation. There can be no methodical science of understanding. Instead, understanding can only ever be produced from a situated, embodied perspective, and the encounter of that situation with a different one. Alongside this, it depends on a fundamental *trust* in the success of dialogue as a way of achieving a 'fusion' of horizons, rather than the subordination of one to the other (as happens in the pursuit of the 'innocent' knowledge that Rossiter refers to). Hence, we can describe Gadamer's ideas as a 'hermeneutics of trust': it focuses on the fundamental relational character of our being, and our understanding in general.

Of course, Gadamer's dialogical model is an ideal scenario. There are times when we fall back into our own horizon and treat interlocutors as 'objects' without their own horizon. We can assume a meaning to their actions and speech based on our own generalisations and stereotypes. Conversely, there is a well-known *doxa* within social work practice that a worker can only 'understand' the situation of a client if they have themselves experienced the problems that the client has (Smith 2008: 3). Within both sets of claims, there is a deliberate distancing of interpreter and interpreted. If we appropriate everything into our own horizon, or insist that meaningful dialogue depends upon a shared perspective or set of experiences, then we would really only be seeing everything as we expect to see it. But in such cases, we cannot say that 'understanding' has taken place; any claim to have the 'final word' on the meaning of experience ignores the ways in which meanings grow and change as the world moves around them. Instead, understanding depends on an open-ness to others, based on the inevitable incompletion of our own knowledge (and, importantly, theirs as well). Rossiter argues that in a social work context 'openness to revelation will [...] require that we practice without allowing the "answer" to dominate the value of the question' (2001: 992). But likewise, attempting to reconstruct the original horizon in its entirety – that is, being completely 'open' to the voice of the other – is similarly futile, for this would empty the message of any significance for us. If our minds were completely 'open', then we would have no way of beginning the dialogue in the first place – we have to anticipate at least part of it. Thus Gadamer argues that the task of hermeneutics 'shows a meaning that claims our attention by addressing it in a manner relevant to our concern with our particular situation' (Hoy 1982: 67). Gadamer's hermeneutics is thus neither restorative (aimed at simply following the clues back to the original meaning of the speaker), nor relativist (remaining within the reader's horizon and disregarding the original meaning). It depends, rather, on the cohesion of dialogue as the formation of speculative understanding.

The hermeneutic circle: anticipating knowledge and reflection

This, of course, involves already committing to dialogue, without necessarily knowing the outcome of it. This means, somewhat paradoxically, we must already be in the process of understanding before we know if we've understood or not. This is known as the hermeneutic circle. Originally described in terms of reading – to understand the sentences in the book, you need to know what the book is 'about'; but to know what it is about, you need to read the sentences in the book – it guides the fundamentally dialogical basis of Gadamer's hermeneutics: 'we must understand the whole in terms of the detail and the detail in terms of the whole' (Gadamer 2004: 291).

We have discussed this so far in terms of an actual dialogue between social worker and service user. But Gadamer uses dialogue primarily as a *metaphor* for understanding, which doesn't limit all of our understanding to actual conversation. How, then, does his claim that interpretation is ontological fit within the broader scope of knowledge-bases for practice?

The idea of what 'understanding' is within social work is often defined through two contrasting approaches: empirically-driven evidence-based practice on the one hand, and the reflective tradition on the other (Healy 2005: 97). It may seem, initially, that Gadamer's account of interpretation keeps us solely in the reflective domain, which runs counter to those calling for a more scientific and evidence-based approach to practice. Historically, professionals have either used scientific method for *conducting* their activities, or used scientific knowledge to *inform* those activities (Kirk and Reid 2002: 115). The latter approach is the form through which social work employed 'science' up to the mid-twentieth century: as a series of models to draw on, separate from the actual application in the field. But empirical research in the 1960s and 1970s into the effectiveness of such uses, in terms of the success of social work interventions, threw up a number of worrying results. Hence, Kirk and Reid argue that this use of objective knowledge to inform practice has occurred at the expense of the former. The lack of objective methodologies to ensure the quality of processes leads to a state where, they argue, 'knowledge' has developed within social work as 'ill-defined and difficult to identify'. As a result, much of social work knowledge has developed without (and shown no active interest in) 'rigorous scientific testing' within social work (2002: 20). Partly, Kirk and

Reid suggest, this is because the use of knowledge to inform, rather than conduct, practice, is dependent upon a knowledge 'infrastructure' (researchers, funding, teaching, textbooks and so on), which is often beyond the control or jurisdiction of practice in itself.

While this criticism is clearly intended to inspire a turn towards a more rigorous and objective approach to usable knowledge, it in fact raises the problem of what social work knowledge actually *is*; and it is this question, I think, that Gadamer's work really addresses. For example, is there a difference between the knowledge-*base* of the profession, and the knowledge of the *effectiveness* of certain practices (which implies an evaluative element based in part on the identity of the profession itself, that as a result goes beyond simple recourse to 'scientific testing' (see Mullen and Streiner 2004))? Are there arch-principles of social work practice that establish certain parameters of flexible and working knowledge within it? Are these principles epistemological, or moral, or constructed from the technical apparatus of 'key institutional and service discourses' (Healy 2005: 194)? As these – distinctly hermeneutic – questions mount up, it is little wonder, then, that Webb argues convincingly a simple recourse to 'evidence' carries with it 'a particular view of human agency and thereby the nature of social work' (2001: 61). No less than any other profession, 'knowledge' within social work has always been a primarily *cultural* issue – that is, an issue embedded within value-laden practices – over and above an epistemological one.

In this sense, the hermeneutic circle alerts us to the point that 'knowledge *of*' something is always and already 'knowledge *for*' something.[4] For this reason, hermeneutics should not be seen as overtly 'reflective', at the expense of its inherent *anticipation* of future understanding. If facts are always integrated into interpretative practices of some kind, then understanding must be circular rather than linear. In Graham Ward's words:

> Interpretations cannot explain; they point to shared, intersubjective meanings and beliefs about what is true, what is real. […] The event or text for which explanation is being sought is transformed by the very act of engagement, and both event and interpretative engagement with it are affected because both participate in wider cultural transformations. (Ward 2005: 69)

Any practice which centres on interpretation is not simply interested in these complex and competing perspectives for its own sake, but rather how questions of norms, power, authority, identity (in all its forms and shapes) get, in the words of David Jardine, 'sorted out, and by whom, and to what end, and so on' (2012: 8). The immediate question that follows any 'making sense' is *to what end* sense has been made. And indeed, from its beginnings, social work knowledge has been invested in the politics of meaning: the very language of 'casework' of the COS was deliberately angled to reflect a systematic approach to poverty (Pierson 2011: 24); the formation of a formal social work education (rather than an on-site apprenticeship) was developed in the United Kingdom in response to reasons ranging from 'immunisation' from the demoralising climate social workers were operating within in, a need to 'prevent internal mental conflicts' (Marshall 1946, quoted in Jones 1996: 192), to supporting the possibility of state social work (Jones 1996: 193); from overcoming its charitable status and becoming a full profession through the adoption of the social and cultural capital of professional status. In all cases, the interpretative ground from which social work knowledge is *produced*, is distinct from knowledge *itself* (be it 'scientific' or 'reflective').

The hermeneutics of suspicion: Jürgen Habermas

But if 'knowledge of' is always 'knowledge for', then the natural question arises: for whom, or for what? This underlies a significant criticism of Gadamer's argument. On the one hand, Gadamer's approach unpacks the relationship between interpretation and understanding, based on the fundamental trust at work in the 'fusion' of horizons. It gives a working sense of the balance required between being open to an other's horizon, and the knowledge, language and prejudices of our own horizons which brings us to be listening to the other in the first place. On the other hand, his work has been criticised on several key points. His emphasis on 'trust' perhaps reflects a model of dialogue too idealistic to fit actual conversations (Billig 1996). Somewhat surprisingly, Gadamer has very little to say about communication where such 'good will' is not present. How would a social worker claim to 'understand' a service user who withholds information, or refuses to cooperate, perhaps on the basis of a deep-rooted mistrust of the social work profession (perceiving that the social worker is there to take away their children, for example)? Gadamer is less clear on this, arguing that this either removes the possibility of understanding (there is no 'real' dialogue to be had), or suggesting that we only identify the lack of dialogue based on a shared understanding of what a real dialogue would look like. In other words, the service user is only able to deceive because they know what a truthful discourse looks like; and, perhaps, they only come into contact with the social worker because of the potential for understanding to occur. This, Gadamer argues, affirms his theory rather than disproves it (2004: 375, n.40).

But in doing so, Gadamer does not discuss the impact of power relations on dialogical understanding. Similarly, he has been criticised for too readily accepting the primacy of 'tradition', and for lacking a critical element at all which would arise from a more defined social and/or cultural dimension. While Gadamer's philosophy was pivotal in developing the primacy of interpretation within culture and society, he himself did not develop its political dimensions at all (Vattimo and Zabala 2011: 77). This absence has led to major critiques emerging from two otherwise opposing sides: the views of Marxist critical theory, voiced through the work of Jürgen Habermas; and the deconstructionist approach of Jacques Derrida. While different in method, both can be identified as following hermeneutics of *suspicion*. We will discuss Derrida's work in more detail in Chapter 5; so for now, we will focus on Habermas's critique.[5]

Habermas agrees with Gadamer's critique of unreflective or positivistic claims to 'meaning', as can be found in some of the more ardently empirical social sciences (Habermas 1988: 153-4). He disagrees, however, that the idea of 'trust' in Gadamer's model of interpretation exists ontologically prior to the interpretation itself. He argues that understanding is not, as Gadamer claims, an act of *being*, but rather is an act of *consciousness*. For Habermas, our consciousness is formed not by tradition in general, but by a *specific* form of tradition, which is ideology. While ideology is often overwhelming (hence, we do not recognise the ideological nature of our understanding of the world), it is possible, at least in theory, to break out from the hermeneutic circle, and to free ourselves from the traditions around us, and to critique our social and cultural practices from the standpoint of *rationality*. Tradition should not be seen as integral to knowledge; rather, it is necessary to suspect and critique the authority upon which tradition is given to us. In this way, Habermas argues, 'Gadamer's prejudice in favour of the legitimacy of prejudices (or prejudgments) validated by tradition is in conflict with the power of reflection, which proves itself in its ability to reject the claim of traditions' (1988: 170). It is precisely the traditions that Gadamer sees as essential to understanding which exclude minority groups and marginalised voices.

Habermas is also critical of what he sees as Gadamer's over-emphasis on language as the arbiter of reality, at the expense of other aspects. Specifically, Habermas argues that there are instead three elements to this: interaction (which Gadamer focuses on), labour and domination. Tradition is therefore more than simply a history of our interactions with others. As a network of symbols and meanings, tradition is dependent on actual conditions which are more than just structures of symbols. Therefore, the purpose of ideology critique is to see through the illusion of our horizons to the reality behind it. Whereas Gadamer's notion of horizon sought to remove the idea of 'innocent' knowledge that was not rooted in one perspective or another, Habermas accuses Gadamer of replacing this with an equally 'innocent' account of horizon. It follows that dialogue and the 'fusion of horizons' cannot be *all* there is to understanding and interpretation. There must be more points of evidence, more spaces for criticism, and more opportunities to challenge the traditions that shape the language we use.

Lovat and Gray argue this aligns Habermasian values with the core of social work:

> It is through the process of coming to know self, invariably entailing an agonizing struggle, that one gradually strips away the inherited knowledge, the familial and cultural baggage, and the ignorance that is so often the source of relational misunderstanding, bigotry, hatred and violence. (Lovat and Gray 2008: 1105)

Unlike Gadamer's sense of tradition, which is fundamentally enabling, Lovat and Gray begin from the broken and dysfunctional relations that social work is often called to address. As Houston notes, service users may have 'experienced debilitating forms of misrecognition', and in such cases it is political critique and self-advocacy that allow individuals to recover their moral worth (Houston 2013: 73–75). In such cases, overcoming 'relational misunderstanding' requires a normative position 'outside' of the tradition from which we speak, or from which we understand ourselves. In Houston's words, the work of Habermas, and the Frankfurt School he was part of, 'needs to be heard more clearly [in social work] as it foregrounds the role of human agency, emotion, critical reflection and their connection with emancipatory action in combating nefarious ideologies' (Houston 2013: 65).

The question then arises, though: what does Habermas base his model of interpretation on, if not tradition? The answer is 'communicative rationality'. For Habermas, both modern scientific and social knowledge have come, in the period of modernity, to utilise only 'instrumental' rationality. As such, this knowledge ceased to have any *critical* role in the value or purpose of such rationality, and ultimately only served to reinforce the status quo. To challenge this, our reasoning and communication – and thus our interpretation – must be based on the possibility of an 'ideal speech situation' where the governing ideologies or traditions that shape our interpretations are no longer in play.

This ideal situation is created through the realisation of consensus. For Habermas, every genuine attempt to communicate involves an attempt to create consensus, as this is the basis of any further interlocution. The dominance of instrumental reason, which Habermas sees as governing modern society – bureaucratic, targets-driven managerialism, for example – is a false form of Enlightenment, corrected only by insisting on the dialogical and consensual nature of societal development. The best way to arrive at such a consensus is the kind of universal rationality that Kant opposed to instrumental reason in his 'What is Enlightenment?' essay, which we discussed in the Introduction to this book. Just as Kant argued that true thinking was thinking for the world, rather than an individual purpose or instrumental goal, so Habermas claims 'that we can know […] proposals for society are rational because they are what we would all choose if we were willing to communicate rationally with each other' (Raffel 1991: 1). In this sense, the ideal speech situation both reflects the conditions by which communication happens at all, and encourages communication beyond the confines of social identity.

In social work, this might be seen in terms of the decisions that a social worker reaches regarding the best intervention strategy. Using the example of children's social work, Spratt and Houston suggest that Habermas's interpretative approach allows social work to engage with governing ideologies – whether they be penal, medical, bureaucratic or other – without becoming subservient to them. Communicative reason requires a re-focus on the essential relationship at the centre of any interpretative work, and this, they argue, allows social workers to re-articulate the terms of assessment: situations dictated as 'risks' by the governing ideology can be recognised as situations of 'problem' or 'need' (1999: 322). Thus, its importance lies in the fact that 'while it does not *remove* the power dimension, the ideal speech situation creates the *possibility* of decisions not merely reflecting pre-held positions' (1999: 320, my emphasis).

> **Thinking through Practice**
>
> Is there such a thing as a decision made that does not reflect pre-held positions? Would it necessarily be beneficial to your practice?
> Which of the models of interpretation – restoration, trust and suspicion – do you most utilise in your own work? Are some more appropriate to specific contexts?

The problem of critique

The issue that began with Gray and Webb's brief definition of interpretation as central to social work practice now seems to rest on the question of critique. While both the hermeneutics of trust and the hermeneutics of suspicion are clear that interpretative acts go on at every level, they differ on whether there is any space *outside* of interpretation from which one can affirm a clear and authentic critical identity.

Gadamer's philosophy questions the assumptions behind what I earlier referred to as an 'instrumental' account of interpretation, and his critique of restorative hermeneutics dismisses the idea that 'meaning' resides solely in the intention of the speaker. Instead, the hermeneutic aspect of knowledge concerns a more fundamental anticipation of an event, an open-ness to the meaning of that event, a vulnerability to the possibilities of the event and its impact on our own horizons. Despite the work that has followed him, Gadamer always insisted that he was not providing a 'method' (2004: 295; the title of his most influential work, *Truth and Method*, was certainly ironic in this respect). Interpretation is not something that we choose, or utilise, but rather something that constitutes our very being. We exist because we interpret. Consequently, there is no 'final interpretation' through which, if the method is followed correctly, the truth will come to be revealed. Meaningfulness 'involves residing (albeit temporarily) in a junction between hermeneutic horizons' (Davey 2006: 198). Because interpretation (and thus understanding) arises from the fusion of different perspectives, it is necessarily dynamic and changing. Indeed, the very conception of 'social work' as a single occupation resides in the historical traditions of what it has been, as well as projections of what it might yet become.

But how might such changes and dynamics occur? For Habermas, traditions must be open to criticism beyond their encounters with other horizons. Interpretation must not trust blindly, but rather *suspect*, given that our traditions are often built upon the exclusion of certain perspectives, and the domination of others. Gadamer's trust in dialogical interaction as the basis of all understanding can be seen as naïve, if, as Habermas argues, it cannot account for other areas of effective knowledge such as labour and domination. There is not much point in transforming lives if no attention is paid to the pre-linguistic limits on such transformation.

Let's consider one final defence of Gadamer's position. In basing his critique upon the idea of the communicative conditions of rationality, Habermas invokes an ideal speech situation that does not, and may never yet, exist. For Vattimo and Zabala, this ideal is only another assertion of something which is beyond critique itself. In this sense, they argue that it is Gadamer's theory which 'is more of a "critical theory" than the work of the Frankfurt School, since it does not need to ground its critical function on metaphysical ideals' (Vattimo and Zabala 2011: 76). Similarly, Graham Ward, whose theory of cultural hermeneutics attempts to develop Gadamer's views in terms of the power relations embedded within our horizons, suggests that the perceived difference between critical theory and hermeneutics is misleading. Whereas the former focuses on 'power, domination, ideology and the production of illusion' – and hence speaks more readily to radical and critical social work contexts – the latter is concerned with 'reference, sense and meaning' (Ward 2005: 62). However, Ward suggests that the critical moment essential to Habermas's ideas is 'only made possible on the basis of a prior act of interpretation'. He continues:

> There can be no critical intervention with respect to a discursive practice without first an evaluation of what is being communicated, inferred, presupposed, etc., in that practice. These evaluations embody modes of interpretation – they practice a hermeneutics even if they do not go on to systematise those modes of interpretation [...] (Ward 2005: 62)

Consequently, Ward argues that the lack of attention paid to the interpretative practices which *underlie critique itself* gives rise to the perception of a 'position' from which critical theory speaks; conversely, hermeneutics appears to not be able to hold such a position, other than its existing traditions, and lacks any political dimensions. But this 'position' appears only because being silent about interpretative practices 'can make critical intervention appear to be a dogmatic truth-claim [...] that cannot itself be negotiated, criticised, refined or denied' (Ward 2005: 62). In other words, if Gadmer's hermeneutics suppresses the power relations within its use of tradition and horizon, critical theory's claim to a 'position' of opposition is, in turn, made only on the back of its suppression of its interpretative practices. The problem, in short, is on what ground Habermas presupposes his ideal consensus takes place, in two senses: first, how he guarantees that such consensus is not itself an act of deprecation or violence; second, whether we can assume that practice-based scenarios, such as that which Spratt and Houston discuss, would in fact make any sense, or have any meaning, in the unconstrained rational scene Habermas imagines.

Nevertheless, the critique of interpretation as a reflection of ideology that Habermas puts forward does bring attention to the notion of *production*. For both Gadamer and Habermas, interpretation takes place within a field of production: for Habermas, this is a field dominated by ideological apparatus that must be resisted and rethought, whereas for Gadamer there is a constantly re-emerging and re-producing ground, which each interpretation challenges to widen and retract.

> **Thinking through Practice**
>
> To what extent do you agree with the claim that interpretation is at the centre of social work practice? Or is there something else at its basis, which interpretation serves? What might it be?

Notes

1 http://www.theguardian.com/uk-news/2014/aug/10/police-right-to-see-medical-records (accessed 16/08/2014).
2 For Furman *et al.*, such commitments 'become the building blocks for practice wisdom that may inform social work practice perhaps even more than research or theory [...] and become woven into the fabric of the profession. Concepts imbedded into current practice wisdom become essential notions related to the human condition and focus practice interventions on resolving various social and psychosocial problems' (Furman *et al.* 2014: 74).
3 Ricoeur specifically states that the former lends itself to therapeutic practices, whereby an original 'reality' is restored; the latter to a psychoanalytic approach whereby an underlying meaning is wrested from an event.
4 This point can often be framed within social sciences as the difference between 'fact' and 'value'. Early thinkers such as Durkheim and Marx tended to see facts (the material or economic conditions of a situation) as determining values: culture could be explained by reference to a 'science' or system of knowledge. Later work by Weber, and more recently the Critical Theory of Habermas, tends to see fact and value as separate spheres. For the *Lebensphilosophie* of Dilthey (and the hermeneutic tradition that followed), values determine the nature of facts. See Lash 1999: 116–123; Gray and Webb 2013: 6.
5 We are focusing here on Habermas's specific critique of Gadamer's hermeneutics; this is obviously not the space for a full analysis of Habermas's full philosophy, or its impact on social work; in particular, the interesting debates between Stan Houston and Paul Michael Garrett on the use of Habermasian frameworks (see Houston 2010).

References

Adams, R., Dominelli, L., and Payne, M. (2009). 'Concluding Comment.' In Adams, R., Dominelli, L., and Payne, M. (eds.), *Practising Social Work in a Complex World*. 2nd edn. Basingstoke: Palgrave Macmillan, pp. 331–5.
Billig, M. (1996). *Arguing and Thinking: A Rhetorical Approach to Social Psychology*. Cambridge: Cambridge University Press.
Burkitt, I. (2008). *Social Selves: Theories of Self and Society*. 2nd edn. London: Sage.
Davey, N. (2006). *Unquiet Understanding*. New York: SUNY Press.
Ferguson, I. and Woodward, R. (2009). *Radical Social Work in Practice: Making a Difference*. Bristol: Policy Press.
Folgheraiter, F. (2004). *Relational Social Work*, A. Belton (trans.). London: Jessica Kingsley Publishers.
Fook, J. (2002). *Social Work: Critical Theory and Practice*. London: Sage.
Furman, R., Enterline, M. D., Lamphear, G. and Shukraft, A. E. (2014). 'Meaning as a Core Principle in Social Work Practice.' *Comunitania: International Journal of Social Work and Social Sciences*, 8, 73–85.

Gadamer, H-G. (2004). *Truth and Method,* J. Weinsheimer (trans.). London: Continuum.
Gray, M., and Webb, S. (2013). 'Introduction.' In Gray, M. and Webb, S. (eds.), *Social Work Theories and Methods.* London: Sage, pp. 1–10.
Habermas, J. (1988). *On the Logic of the Social Sciences,* S. Weber Nicholsen and J. Stark (trans.). Cambridge, MA: MIT Press.
Harrison, G. (2009). 'Language Politics, Linguistic Capital and Bilingual Practitioners in Social Work.' *British Journal of Social Work,* 39, 1082–100.
Healy, K. (2005). *Social Work Theories in Context: Creating Frameworks for Practice.* Basingstoke: Palgrave Macmillan.
Heritage, J. (1984). *Garfinkel and Ethnomethodology.* Englewood Cliffs, NJ: Prentice-Hall.
Hirsch, E. (1967). *Validity in Interpretation.* New Haven, CT: Yale University Press.
Hoy, D. (1982). *The Critical Circle: Literature, History and Philosophical Hermeneutics.* London: University of California Press.
Houston, S. (2010). 'Further Reflections on Habermas' Contribution to Discourse in Child Protection: An Examination of Power in Social Life.' *British Journal of Social Work,* 40 (6).
—— (2013). 'Social Work and the Politics of Recognition.' In Gray, M. and Webb, S. (eds.), *The New Politics of Social Work.* Basingstoke: Palgrave Macmillan, pp. 63–76.
Humphreys, R. (1995). *Sin, Organised Charity and the Poor Law in Victorian England.* London: St. Martin's Press.
Jardine, D. (2012). 'The Descartes Lecture'. *Journal of Applied Hermeneutics.* Available at: http://www.academia.edu/7934509/The_Descartes_Lecture.
Jones, C. (1996). 'Anti-Intellectualism and the Peculiarities of British Social Work Education.' In Parton, N. (ed.), *Social Theory, Social Change and Social Work.* London: Routledge, pp. 190–210.
Kirk, S., and Reid, W. (2002). *Science and Social Work: A Critical Appraisal.* New York: Columbia University Press.
Lash, S. (1999). *Another Modernity, A Different Rationality.* Oxford: Blackwell.
Lipsky, M. (1980). *Street-Level Bureaucrats: The Dilemmas of Individuals in Public Service.* New York: Russell Sage Foundation.
Lovat, T., and Gray, M. (2008). 'Towards a Proportionist Social Work Ethics: A Habermasian Perspective.' *British Journal of Social Work,* 38, 1100–14.
Lymbery, M. (2005). *Social Work with Adults.* London: Sage.
Lynton, E. (1990). 'New Concepts of Professional Expertise: Liberal Learning as Part of Career-oriented Education.' *Resource Centre for Higher Education,* Boston, MA. Available at: http://eric.ed.gov/ERICDocs/data/ericdocs2sql/content_storage_01/0000019b/80/12/fc/7f.pdf
McBeath, G. and Webb, S. (2002). 'Virtue Ethics and Social Work: Being Lucky, Realistic and Not Doing One's Duty.' *British Journal of Social Work,* 32, 1015–36.
McLaughlin, H. (2012). *Understanding Social Work Research.* 2nd edn. London: Sage.
Moules, N., McCaffrey, G., Morck, A. and Jardine, D. (2011). 'Editorial: On Applied Hermeneutics and the Work of the World.' *Journal of Applied Hermeneutics,* 1, 1–5.
Mullen, E.J. and Streiner, D. L. (2004). 'The Evidence For and Against Evidence-Based Practice.' *Brief Treatment and Crisis Intervention,* 4, 2, 111–21.
Pierson, J. (2011). *Understanding Social Work: History and Context.* Maidenhead: Open University Press.
Preston-Shoot, M. (2007). 'Whose Lives and Whose Learning? Whose Narratives and Whose Writing? Taking the Next Research and Literature Steps with Experts by Experience.' *Evidence & Policy,* 3, 3, 343–59.
Raffel, S. (1991). *Habermas, Lyotard and the Concept of Justice.* Basingstoke: Macmillan Academic and Professional.

Ricoeur, P. (1970). *Freud and Philosophy: An Essay on Interpretation*, D. Savage (trans.). New Haven, CT: Yale University Press.
Rossiter, A. (2001). 'Innocence Lost and Suspicion Found: Do we Educate For or Against Social Work?' *Critical Social Work*, 2, 1. Available at http://www1.uwindsor.ca/criticalsocialwork/innocence-lost-and-suspicion-found-do-we-educate-for-or-against-social-work
Schleiermacher, F. (1998). *Hermeneutics and Criticism and Other Writings*. Ed. Andrew Bowie. Cambridge: Cambridge University Press.
Scourfield, P. (2010). 'A Critical Reflection on the Involvement of "Experts by Experience" in Inspections.' *British Journal of Social Work*, 40, 1890–907.
Searle, J. (1979). *Expression and Meaning: Studies in the Theory of Speech Acts*. Cambridge: Cambridge University Press.
—— (1993). 'Metaphor.' In Ortony, A. (ed.), *Metaphor and Thought*. Cambridge: Cambridee University Press, pp. 83–111.
Smith, R. (2008). *Social Work and Power*. Basingstoke: Palgrave Macmillan.
Spratt, T. and Houston, S. (1999). 'Developing Critical Social Work in Theory and in Practice: Child Protection and Communicative Reason.' *Child and Family Social Work*, 4, 315–24.
Teater, B. (2010). *An Introduction to Applying Social Work Theories and Methods*. Maidenhead: Open University Press.
Vattimo, G. and Zabala, S. (2011). *Hermeneutic Communism: From Heidegger to Marx*. New York: Columbia University Press.
Ward, G. (2005). *Cultural Transformation and Religious Practice*. Cambridge: Cambridge University Press.
Webb, S. (2001). 'Some Considerations on the Validity of Evidence-based Practice in Social Work.' *British Journal of Social Work*, 31, 57–79.
White, S. and Stancombe, J. (2002). 'Colonising Care? Potentialities and Pitfalls of a Scientific-Bureaucratic Rationality in Social Care.' *Journal of Social Work Research and Evaluation*, 3, 2, 187–202.
Woodcock Ross, J. (2011). *Specialist Communication Skills for Social Workers*. Basingstoke: Palgrave Macmillan.

2
COMMUNITY

The case of the missing community

Community: ever more significant?

Both Gadamer's and Habermas's accounts of interpretation require thinking through the ways in which meaning is mediated by our relation to others. By challenging the objectivist insistence on a strict separation between interpreter and interpreted, they raise questions regarding the *communal basis* of our knowledge. The question of community, like the question of interpretation, offers a key area of intersection between social work and philosophy. While community practice has always been fundamental to social work since its earliest days (Dominelli 2004), it has always been accompanied by disputed claims over the nature of its work, class, identity and purpose. What actually *constitutes* the community is a continuously contested topic, and one which has important implications for how social work situates itself in relation to the increasingly politicised use of 'community' as not only a set of relations between people, but also as a symbol of cultural practices and traditions. As such, the question of what the basis of community is challenges both social work and philosophy alike.

If the pluralist nature of contemporary society is often illustrated through the term 'community' – that is, society is made up of a range of different cultures and communities – it is also, itself, a pluralist concept, invoking a range of different and often conflicting meanings. 'Community work' can refer not only to ground-up social work practices, but also to punitive sentences for young offenders (Garland 2001); 'the community' can refer to an inclusive sense of shared place, meaning and value (Powell and Geoghegan 2004), as well as an exclusive boundary around particular groups based on particular attributes, such as ethnicity. Indeed, the notion of community within social work – whether as 'community social work' itself, typically located in the voluntary sector; or as the 'community development and social action' that radical social work opposed to the perceived pathologising of individualist casework (Lymbery 2005: 47); or the community as an affective term within statutory social work – is often problematised by the political initiatives which surround and shape it (Rose 1996; Pavelová 2014). Increasingly, 'community development is under siege as a process-oriented, contextually sensitive means of promoting participation in civil society and politics', argues Mary Lane. 'Agendas are handed down with funding packages […] and emphasis is on predefined goals rather than on accounts of lived experience' (1999: 146). In broader sociological terms, Price and Simpson note that in recent years there has been 'an increased emphasis upon community within social work, at a time when the ways in which people relate to one another are being increasingly individualised and decreasingly collective' (2007: 136).

This dual sense of the community, as both fundamentally important and inherently contested, often circulates around the sense that the community is not-quite-present: whether this is in terms of a nostalgic yearning for a lost community (for example, Schirmer and Michailakis 2015); or the representation of a group that sits 'outside' of mainstream discussion and policy-making (for example, the 'Muslim community', the 'deaf community', etc.); or in respect to the relative lack of interest amongst social work students in engaging with community practice (Koeske *et al.* 2005); and the perceived need to recover social work's interest in community contexts as a counterpoint to its focus on interpersonal and family networks (Lynn 2006). Zygmunt Bauman once claimed that community is something we 'miss'; and in all these cases, we can read this in two ways: it seems that we not only miss the *memory* of community, but also miss it in the sense of talking over it or around it, whilst failing to articulate its core principles.

Thinking through Practice

Is it possible to formulate a clear definition of what kind of community you live, practice or work within? What is this definition based on – geographical location? Shared activities? Something else?

Despite this, the term 'community' remains, in Christopher Fynsk's terms, an 'imperative'. Like the often-accompanying notion of 'freedom', 'community' still speaks to us with a sense of demand: 'even if political discourses have proven unable to give them a meaning that *holds* for a social practice devoted to socio-political needs, we find ourselves unable to do without them, even haunted by them in some sense' (Fynsk 1991: ix). Jean-Luc Nancy thus begins his essay on *The Inoperative Community* in a sombre tone:

> The gravest and most painful testimony of the modern world, the one that possibly involves all other testimonies to which this epoch must answer […] is the testimony of the dissolution, the dislocation, or the conflagration of community. (1991: 1)

How should we conceive of community specifically in terms of this sense of both demand and loss, and in terms of the ambiguity over the meaning and significance of community itself? In this chapter, I want to examine the dominant philosophical attempts to answer this question of what community is, which have been mainly shaped by the debate between liberal and communitarian viewpoints. While both highlight a 'missing' sense of community that resonates with the contestations mentioned above, both can be critiqued for under-examining the vitality of the interpersonal relations central to social work practice. The work of Nancy, meanwhile, suggests a different sense in which the community can be said to be missed: that attempts to present a unified or reductive sense of what a community 'is' paradoxically undermine the very sociality that brings people together in the first place.

Community, society and modernity

Arguments over the nature of what a community is, or should be, go back to the ancient philosophers: Plato's *Republic*, Thucydides' *Melian Dialogue*, Aristotle's *Politics* and *Nichomachean Ethics*, and so on. But it was in the nineteenth century, at the same time as modern social work was first forming, that philosophical ideas were exchanged regarding the contrast between communal gathering and solidarity, and the wider movements of the newly-defined 'society'. Some, such as the work of Hegel and Schelling, were concerned with what we might broadly call the philosophy of history: that is, ideas as to how and why change occurred from the earliest communities to the present, how they developed and whether they progressed in line with the human capacity to think and will. For others, this development was acutely tied, dialectically, to European industrialisation and the growth of liberal economics. Ferdinand Tönnies, for example, argued that community (*Gemeinschaft*) was an 'ideal type' of social relationship, formed by the human will (Tönnies 2003: 103). The will to be part of a community was based on a 'natural' will to act in accordance with the general ends of the group. Such a natural will was based on three elements: kinship (the connection to others through family relationships), locality (the connection to a particular area over a period of time), and mind (the connection to those with shared ideas). As an ideal type, the principles of community were not necessarily 'real' in an immediate sense, but presupposed by the actions of the individuals within the community (Price and Simpson 2007: 117). *Gemeinschaft* operated at the level of family, village or town: small groups which were increasingly challenged by both the rise of increased communications, transport and social mobility, and the decline of shared cultural values and moral codes. As such, Tönnies argued, modernity saw the rise of society (*Gesellschaft*); which operated according to the rational will. Here, individuals engaged with others in order to achieve their own ends; social relationships were premised on instrumental reason. This, in turn, affected the conditions of the *Gemeinschaft*: rather than the rational will superseding the natural sense of social relations, new forms of community instead emerged in and around the larger entities of the city, the state, the global network that constituted the *Gesellschaft*. Society replaces community, and communities must in turn respond by finding places to re-emerge within society. Here, the very concept of 'community' arises only in terms of its fading significance next to larger, dis-located concepts of social grouping.

> **Thinking through Practice**
>
> In an article discussing the use of Tönnies' distinction between society and community for social work education, Jacob Kornbeck argues that '*Gesellschaft* has until now been the predominant mode in both teaching and practice. *Gemeinschaft* is a neglected aspect with considerable potential added-value both for theory and practice' (2001: 259). Using the example of education around immigration and immigrant communities, he suggests that teaching based on *Gesellschaft* would focus on, for example, 'scientific psychology' or 'immigration law courses', whereas a *Gemeinschaft* approach would encourage 'experiencing principles of social interaction' and contributions from members of 'immigrant' communities (258).
>
> But given Tönnies' argument about the disappearance and subsequent re-emergence of *Gemeinschaft* as normative concepts for organising social relations, what are the risks for this approach to social work education?
>
> How easy is it to separate 'society' from 'community', within your own practice and/or learning? On what grounds do you draw that distinction?

As a way of understanding different social relations, Tönnies' distinction between the 'rational and abstract society' and the 'lived and embodied community', as normative concepts, may have since been developed, if not superseded. But it remains useful for clarifying three points for our discussion here.

1. The premise of any community is not necessarily based on an immanent or immediately visible set of social or geographical relations. As Benedict Anderson famously argued (1983), communities are as much about the imagination as they are physical relationships. Often, community is seen as being based on a foundational 'mythology' (see, for example, the anthropological work of Levi-Strauss 1981: 679) which narrates the organisation of its various aspects. So community is, and will always be, tied to the rhetorical projections. And if this leaves it open to manipulation by political interests, it also allows for numerous spaces of resistance to such interests. Hence, Boris Groys (2010) has argued that in the contemporary world of global communications – from telecommunications to the advent of Web 2.0 – new 'communities' can, in principle at least, be founded and dissolved with speed and ease. But at the same time, the governing principles of communal identity have been more glacial in moving. The more common *mythos* of modern community – the clear focal points such as class, race, gender – remain pressing (Featherstone 1995).

2. When this imaginary of the community is challenged by material and economic forces – such as modern industrialisation in the nineteenth century, or the rise of neoliberal economics in the 1970s and 1980s and its effect on social care – this does not directly cause the breakdown of the community. For Tönnies, it is in fact the breakdown of community which *allows* for the idea of society to challenge it in the first place; the dissolving and dis-location (to paraphrase Nancy) of the idea of the community opens up a space for the rational will to emerge, along with the market-driven society that it produces. Because community precedes society, the ideas and imaginary of community remain more persistent than their actual realisation.
3. Tönnies' argument shapes the idea of the community fundamentally around the idea of the self. Community is discussed in terms of how people relate to each other *as separate individuals*, and in what name or image. In this sense, it is indebted to a paradigmatic way of doing political philosophy that assumes we exist as 'individuals' in some ontological or existential way *before* we exist in relation to others. This point is a key differential between the philosophical approaches to community.

These points, first made in the nineteenth century, remain crucial to any consideration of the role of community within social work, because they reflect three fundamental concerns regarding, first, the *ways of thinking* community (that is, the modes of reasoning we apply); second, the *temporality* of community (that is, how it changes and develops over time); and third, the *task or purpose* of community. These three concerns provide a key intersection between philosophical discussions of community, and social work's invocations of community as central to practice.

John Rawls and the liberal community

What conditions, then, should we be looking for when we invoke the idea of 'community'? In the twentieth and twenty-first century, the philosophical question of what the community is has been directed by two dominant arguments. One side can be broadly defined as the 'liberal'[1] approach, characterised by the likes of John Rawls and Robert Nozick; the other side can be termed 'communitarian', represented by thinkers such as Alasdair MacIntyre, Michael Walzer, and Michael Sandel.

The liberal view begins from the idea of a self-interested individual, who relates to other self-interested individuals on the basis of a 'social contract'. Community, and the society surrounding it, thus serves and protects the individual. For Rawls, these ideas revolve around the notion of distributive justice, which concerns how justice is organised according to the distribution of wealth, resource and opportunity within a community or society. When Rawls first published his landmark book *A Theory of Justice* in 1971, it was a response to the dominant utilitarian approach to understandings of community. For utilitarian thinking, the rule of the majority outweighs the minority; what is good for the many is good for society as a whole, and hence individual interests should always be subordinate to the wellbeing of the group as a whole. Contrary to this, Rawls is interested in preserving the dynamic individuality of a community. But, he argues, such differences between people (in terms of morals, religious belief, social practices and so on) must be held together by procedural principles. These principles can only be based on the rights of the individual to carry out their interests, as – given the pluralistic society we live in – it would be impossible to agree on any foundational 'good' for us all to follow. In Rawls' words, 'the concept of right [is] prior to that of the good' (1971: 31). His argument, then, begins by affirming that any bonds of community, and the governing of social relationships, must be *procedural* rather than normative.

Why does Rawls insist on this approach? This needs to be situated in both the conceptual and material effects of the Enlightenment project. Originally, the Enlightenment promised the discovery of universal principles that would determine right from wrong. On this basis, the older governance by tradition and assumed authority could be overthrown. However, when the previous metaphysical certainties and assumed structures that delineated the world are increasingly questioned, the effects are not to dispel *Gemeinschaft*, but rather to encourage new, sometimes competing, and compelling narratives of social relations. As such, society develops pluralistically, driven by and responding to socio-cultural phenomena such as the global movement (or displacement) of populations, the rise of alternative and new mainstream ideologies and moral outlooks, and a range of potentially conflicting narratives and myths of community. This is, of course, reflected in social work practice and education with the pressing centrality of 'culturally competent practice' regarding race, ethnicity, gender, sexuality and so on (see Rothman 2008).

As Virginia Held explains, the assumption of liberal philosophy is that 'in a pluralistic society and even more clearly in a pluralistic world, we cannot agree on our visions of the good life […] but we can hope to agree on the *minimal conditions* for justice, for coexistence within a framework allowing us to pursue our visions of the good life' (Held 1999: 338, my emphasis). Some obvious minimal conditions or foundational principles may come to mind – equality and liberty are usually among the first responses. But equal in what *ways*? At liberty to do *what*? Rawls answers this with his famous thought-experiment of the 'original position'. He asks us to imagine that members of a society are given the opportunity to decide how wealth and power should be distributed. The caveat is that they must do so from behind a 'veil of ignorance' – a hypothetical position whereby nobody knows what role they themselves will have in the society that they are planning. Neither do they know what abilities, physical and mental, they will have. Under such conditions, Rawls argues, participants should choose to divide wealth and power in such a way that opportunity is distributed as equally as possible. It is a bit like baking a cake between five people and deciding on the best way to cut it, without knowing who will get what slice. The rational position would be to divide the cake equally, so that you were ensured getting the best possible slice, rather than cutting one big slice and several small ones, in the hope that you end up with the biggest.

The original position is not supposed to actually take place historically. It is part of a long tradition – a *way of thinking* community – within political philosophy of imagining a space whereby society is created, in order to affirm or critique the organisation of our actual existing society. By reducing the question of community to one basic issue – how best to manage our self-interests in relation to our resources – Rawls suggests that we would rationally agree on certain outcomes, which amount to two specific principles. First, there is a principle of equality: there should be equality in the distribution of basic rights and duties. Everyone should have 'an equal right to the most extensive basic liberty compatible with a similar liberty for others' (Rawls 1971: 60–1). Second, there is the principle of difference: inequality, whether social, economic or moral, is only considered 'just' if it results in compensating benefits for everyone (1971: 302). The first principle effectively curtails the reaches of the second: once everyone is afforded equal rights, this means that the second principle must follow that inequality must be justified in terms of those same rights. Rawls thus argues that the *purpose* of community is to value liberal freedom, while maintaining a duty to the wellbeing of all. Society is 'a cooperative venture for mutual advantage' (Rawls 1971: 4). On this foundation, Rawls suggests we should follow a 'reflective equilibrium' whereby we bring our theoretical sense of justice into balance with our day-to-day practices.

It makes no sense, Rawls argues, to allow inequality to fester uncontrollably until the mass wealth of the few forces the many into deprivation. Thus, in more practical terms, this is a liberal justification for the welfare 'safety net' that exists beneath a free market capitalist society. The reason is that, for Rawls, almost all inequality is fundamentally unjust: someone may have more money than someone else, but this could be due to inheritance. Somebody may work harder than someone else, but this could be due to a particular form of upbringing. A person does not choose to not have learning disabilities, any more than someone who has learning disabilities does. In all cases, an individual's success is always, ultimately, down to chance. Given that our resources and opportunities in life are often due to accidents of birth (wealthy parents, a natural aptitude for high quality work, physical ability, and so on) which we do not ourselves choose, then this cannot and should not figure in the discussion of communal justice (see Dworkin 1981). Rather, the procedural bonds of community must, if anything, compensate for the starting inequality we inevitably find ourselves in by virtue of being different from one another.

Thinking through Practice

To what extent do you find Rawls' justification of equal rights applicable to the ethos of social work practice? Is he correct to approach this commitment to equality as a procedural one, or are there *other* justifications for promoting equality and diversity within society?

Criticisms of the liberal individual

The advent of social, cultural and moral pluralism as a consequence of individual freedom means that Rawls is concerned with justice at the level of societal organisation.

Communities require the minimal conditions of justice laid down *by* society in order to work; but as they are in practice more emotional, historical or intimate relationships, they cannot be seen as the *same thing* as society. This is not to say that the community is not important for Rawls: indeed, late on in *A Theory of Justice* he argues that 'only in social union is the individual complete' (1971: 525), as this provides affirmation of the self through communities of shared interests. However, such communities should be *chosen* rather than assumed. Although Rawls notes that we will always, practically, have some kind of attachment to groups or shared aims (1971: 14), he denies that these should play a role in our philosophising about what constitutes a society. Social unity cannot be based on a shared identity or moral purpose; the pluralistic make-up of our cities, towns, and streets simply does not permit this. Thus, communities reflect societies inasmuch as they are nothing really more than the sum of its parts – a collection of 'unencumbered' individuals.

But we seem to have missed something here, and the more the liberal approach is developed and applied, the more this absence becomes evident. In the work of Robert Nozick, for example, there is an argument that the interests of individual freedom should *always* outweigh those of the state or community. Despite its radical libertarianism, Nozick's work, alongside the economic theories of Friedrich Hayek and Milton Friedman, was hugely influential on the New Right social policies in the 1980s in both the United States and United Kingdom, and helped to lay the foundations for the morphing of liberalist philosophy into neoliberal social policy: a move which brought about the shrinking of state-funded welfare and the introduction of 'marketisation' of social services (see Webb 2006). Social *injustice*, for these thinkers, arose from the interference of any centralised distributor of justice. It was this – the very notion of welfare intervention – which created unjust inequality. Left to our own devices, the rationality of economics was enough to order individuals effectively. Nozick argues that the aim of society, such that it has an aim at all, should be the guaranteeing of a minimal amount of safety and minimal interference in the activities of individuals. Engagement with others, Nozick argues, is always a sacrifice of our individual freedom, and 'there is no justified sacrifice of some of us for others' (Nozick 1974: 33). It is not a far step from this reasoning to Margaret Thatcher's well-known dictum of 1980s social policy in the United Kingdom that 'there is no such thing as society', delivered in an interview with *Woman's Own* magazine in 1987: that people cannot inflict their problems (poverty, homelessness, disability and so on) on society, because 'it's our duty to look after ourselves and then, also to look after our neighbour' (Keay 1987).

I want to briefly note here several important differences between the classical tradition of liberalism, of which Rawls and Nozick form a part, and the neoliberal philosophy which extends more directly from Hayek's work. Wendy Brown notes four such differences (2005: 40):

1. Neoliberalism presumes that economic rationality can be applied to all aspects of human life, not just the economic ones (thus social, cultural and political life is predicated on scarcity of resources).

2. While classical liberalism was *laissez-faire* (if markets were left to themselves, they would naturally balance themselves), neoliberalism requires that the market is 'directed, buttressed, and protected by law and policy as well as by the dissemination of social norms' (41). The health of the economy thus becomes the basis of state legitimacy.
3. Neoliberalism constructs the individual as an 'entrepreneurial actor in every sphere of life' (42), which dramatically changes Rawls' account of the 'free individual' to one who is free in terms of their market capability.
4. Neoliberalism transforms the 'criteria for good social policy' (44) by requiring inequality as a base target for success.

There is a space, then, for Rawls' account of the community to resist the specifically *economic* rationalisation of regulation of social services and social work provision that the neoliberal agenda has ushered in, by emphasising the necessary requirement of welfare in order for a community to exist rationally. At the same time, this argument may still appear to miss something fundamental about community. I mentioned before that community was problematic in terms of three concerns: *thinking*, *temporality* and *purpose*. In this case, I would argue that what is missed, from social work perspectives, is rooted in the mode of thinking Rawls employs.

Because the liberal approach values rational deliberation, it subjects the experiences of community to rational deliberation, as though we can 'step outside' of those experiences and re-constitute them according to rational principles. It is a social contract theory, whereby any communal body is formed on the basis of an implicit or explicit contractual understanding: the giving up of certain freedoms for the gain of certain benefits. But the mode of reasoning also determines the content of the argument. As a result, we are left with an account of community that suggests individuals simply 'appear' in some pre-social space, and then merge together to form a social group. Just as Tönnies did, the liberal approach views the members of a community as being *essentially* individual. This follows a path taken by modern philosophy since Thomas Hobbes suggested that we should 'consider men as if but even now sprung out of the earth, and suddenly, like mushrooms, come to full maturity, without all kind of engagement with each other' (Hobbes 1972: 205). In other words, we should purposefully ignore the *existing* relationships people find themselves in.

The reason that this is significant is primarily how Hobbes proceeds from this suggestion. Hobbes asks us to consider that, without the structures of the state around us, the world would be a 'state of nature'. This is a wild, uncivilised and violently individualistic situation where people wander the world surviving against all others; where life is, famously, 'nasty, brutish and short'. Society would emerge, Hobbes argues, when individuals band together under a social contract, sacrificing some of their individual freedom for the security that greater numbers provide. Rawls' original position can be seen as a highly abstracted version of Hobbes' state of nature. But whereas he avoids Hobbes' more detailed and specific account of what a human being may be before society, the image of the state of nature has remained firmly pressed into the Western imaginary. While originally only ever meant as a thought experiment, such ideas coincided with European expansion into the 'New World' in the sixteenth and seventeenth centuries, where colonists encountered 'natives' who appeared, to the European eye at least, to be enacting the very state Hobbes had described. In this way, the sense of individualism at work in political philosophy has become a curiously quasi-historical entity. It embedded the idea that members of communities are fundamentally in competition with each other, and with other communities. And indeed, the idea that, at heart, we are all animalistic (and, consequently, violent), and society's rules keep us in check and 'civilise' us to forget these base instincts, seems to be confirmed when states dissolve into civil war, when society breaks down due to famine or poverty, or even when a child lashes out at another who has taken their toy. It seems to be supported by numerous experiments in psychology – the Stanford Prison Experiment, for example (Zimbardo 1971). It is, arguably, heavily implied in models such as Maslow's hierarchy of needs (Maslow 1970), that in turn form the basis of 'graded care' for the assessment of service user need (see, for example, Hopkins and Hill 2010), child neglect (see Ayre 2007), or even for healthy management strategies of social workers themselves (see Lewis *et al.* 2001). But all of these are inseparable from a particular cultural *imaginary*, carried within a particular mode of thinking. Separating the reality of such 'findings' from the framing image of the individual is difficult; hence why Hobbes' notion of violence based on scarcity of resources remains convincing, even though 'scarcity' has a very different meaning in today's global north (see Wilkinson 2005: 3–8). Because of this, it is unclear just how 'real' this individual, separable from society by virtue of such reasoning and imagination, actually can be; and, if real at all, whether this is the best person to, in fact, be judging which community is the best.

In attempting to remove the problematic assumptions of Hobbes' state of nature, and so justify a general equality for all, Rawls' rational individual becomes an abstract entity, divorced from its embodiment, social ties, family relations and non-possessive desires. In doing so, it exhibits 'a certain abstract and ghostly character' (MacIntyre 1981: 31) and this surely misses out a key component of the self: that is, the physical and emotional relationships already in existence around it, and the forms through which these relationships are recognised and maintained; what Margaret Lynn refers to as the 'person-in-the-situation' that social work is committed to (2006: 110). It could be argued, then, that what is 'missing' in the liberal account are the layers of capability within the act of reasoning itself; and here the work of Pierre Bourdieu has been hugely instructive, in terms of how the effectiveness of rationality, acting and thinking are conditioned by the value of their capital (see Garrett 2013: 121–149). Bourdieu's work allows us to see that 'the different cultural discourses, and therefore the different forms of *interpretative reasoning*, are not situated upon a level playing field and have on deposit various forms and different amounts of capital' (Ward 2005: 67, my emphasis). If individuals are always born out of and into relationships (whether caring or not), which are cultivated within networks of meaning and value (whether accessible or not), then it makes no sense to imagine that we can reason over the nature of a just society outside of these.

Given that our social, moral and political judgements will all depend on the available language we have to express them, and our predispositions towards certain views over others, it makes no sense to begin thinking about community from the perspective of an abstract individual.

The rise of communitarianism

Alasdair MacIntyre's book *After Virtue* (1981) identified the dominance of liberalism as a problematic base for any coherent and meaningful social norms, and in particular its continuous insistence on the centrality of the individual rational agent over and above their social context. If the liberal self is 'unencumbered', the communitarian self is always *situated*.

Just like Rawls, MacIntyre begins *After Virtue* with a brief thought experiment of his own; or, as he puts it, a 'disquieting suggestion'. He imagines that all of our scientific discoveries gradually disappear. Scientists are dispossessed and cast out of society, and teaching science is banned. Many years later, the fable continues, there is an attempt to revive science. But nobody is around who knows it as it was; and they can only find scraps of paper and fragments of theories: 'a knowledge of experiments detached from any knowledge of the theoretical context which gave them significance' (1981: 1). But these fragments are collected together and established as a thing called 'science'; it is taught in schools and forms the basis of new university departments and intellectual debate. However, without the original experiments to provide any foundation to the debate, inevitably the claim would be made that science was simply a question of how you arranged the fragments you held. It would be what the individual made it to be. This thought experiment is not, of course, about science at all. Rather, MacIntyre argues, this is precisely what *has* happened to the world of ethics. The principles of morality invoked in contemporary social work practice – individual freedom, human rights, empowerment and development – are, MacIntyre would suggest, all lacking the fundamental structure which makes morality *moral*. Furthermore, reconstructing ideas such as 'community', 'care', or 'ethical duty' without their original structure is akin to the new science created in his thought experiment.

He draws on the anthropological work of Mary Douglas on 'taboo' as a further parallel with the case of morality. Douglas suggests that such taboos have two stages of development: in the first stage, they emerge from out of a specific context which makes the ruling of the taboo meaningful. In the second stage, such contexts are lost or forgotten, but the rule itself remains, and is often unable to be explained rationally by those who follow it. 'In such a situation,' MacIntyre relates, 'the rules have been deprived of any status that can secure their authority and, if they do not acquire some new status quickly, both their interpretation and their justification become debatable' (1981: 112). Furthermore, '[w]hen the resources of a culture are too meagre to carry through the task of re-interpretation, the task of justification becomes impossible' (112). He applies this to the case of liberal philosophy: its emphasis on individualism is entirely at odds with the very concepts it uses individualism to justify – justice, equality and so on.

It is no small coincidence that MacIntyre's ideas were also circulating around the time that the use of the term 'community' was increasingly politicised and re-defined in social care contexts.[2] As Price and Simpson document, in the UK the 1980s 'saw a move away from institutional care, prompted by research into its effects and a general lack of efficacy' (2007: 134), leading to the large-scale closure of children's homes, local authority residential homes for the elderly, and changes to the custodial methods of dealing with young offenders, which all placed an emphasis on the 'community' or immediate family and kinship groups. In the UK, the 1990 NHS and Community Care Act saw the state as an 'enabler' rather than a 'provider' of care, with the service user taking on a quasi-customer role once they had been assessed, allowing them to 'purchase' services that, it was suggested, would increasingly come from the wider community rather than the state or institutional care. The problem was that the community remained under-defined throughout: principally, it was referred to only in the sense that 'community care is not institutional care' (Price and Simpson 2007: 133). If such a programme was engendered through familiar liberal language – 'empowerment', 'rights', 'self-realisation' and so on – MacIntyre argues that such terms will remain hopelessly arbitrary *unless* we recognise how our interpretation of them as meaningful at all depends upon a particular set of narratives, which are embedded within our communal traditions (1981: 210). Without this, we are left with what McBeath and Webb refer to as the 'glossy HMSO documents' invoking 'phrases such as "best practice" which reflect "inclusivist" ideas of participation', but mediated through the 'post-Thatcherite political language of [...] public ethics' (2002: 1019–20). In short, community has to be re-appropriated, outside of the modern liberal norms that had confused its meaning.

To do this, MacIntyre proposes that small-scale communities, linked through shared notions of the common good, are the only way to ensure the continuation of social bonds and morality. Not just any community will do, however: there are three aspects in particular which he argues are necessary for a flourishing moral community – practice, narrative and moral tradition – that can effectively combat the problems of liberal individualism:

Practice. We become better people through social practices. Practices are 'any coherent and complex form of socially established cooperative human activity' that enables 'goods internal to that form of activity' to be realised in the course of achieving the 'standards of excellence which are appropriate to, and partially definitive of, that form of activity' (MacIntyre 1981: 187). In short, social practices are formed through the roles that we play within a given group or community: parent, carer, bus driver and so on. Each of these roles has an accompanying sense of 'practical wisdom' as to how the roles are best performed. Hence, social practices can be said to have 'virtues' which we practise both to develop our own abilities, and to know if we're getting better at them.

Narrative. We can't simply apply virtues, like we do rules, to individual situations, as Rawls attempts with his overarching definition of 'justice'. Being 'good' is something we learn, and, hopefully, get better at: in turn, so does the community around us. McBeath and Webb argue similarly that social work practice should be seen as 'dispositional' rather than 'functional'; and that social work 'should recognise that moral agents are constituted by a play of forces which shape the capacity for good (or bad) judgement and action' (2002: 1016). MacIntyre thus argues we must understand the individual within a narrative framework: the self is an unfolding story that is yet to be finished.

Moral tradition. This narrative is determined by the traditions we are part of. What it is to be 'good' or 'virtuous' is embedded within the history of those traditions. Without these, we would not be able to measure how 'good' our actions were. What we lose when 'community' becomes an empty or fragmented term, MacIntyre argues, is a sense of a unifying goal that brings people together, and directs their practices as a group.

In other words, it is precisely what Rawls removed from his philosophy of community – that is, any sense of shared purpose beyond its basic procedural elements (see Rawls 1985: 249) – that MacIntyre wants to reinstate. To use our earlier vocabulary, the *task* of community dictates the *ways of thinking* about it. Without these shared goals and purposes, any disagreement between individuals on moral issues becomes separated from factual content. Without the construction of 'local forms of community within which civility and the intellectual and moral life can be sustained' (MacIntyre 1981: 262), we are left with 'interminable debates' regarding what is right and wrong, and we are reduced to simply a case of shouting at each other until one person gives in.

> **Thinking through Practice**
>
> MacIntyre is notoriously quiet on what such communities would actually be; though groups such as parent/teacher associations, or directorial boards of hospitals, are sometimes given as examples. What kind of 'small communities with shared goals' might be relevant to social work practice, and in what ways might their shared goals help in clarifying the role of that community?

Radical future, or nostalgic ideal?

Is MacIntyre's communitarianism a radical re-envisioning of community, capable of genuine change in people's lives, or is it simply regretting the loss of a once-coherent sense of belonging in a now incoherent world? Certainly, it relies on a sense of community which is *both* in the past, *and* yet to be realised. We cannot discuss community, MacIntyre suggests, without getting right to the bottom of why it seems so difficult to identify or conceptualise. Hence, he diagnoses the problems of modern thinking, and in particular its emphasis on the rational individual, as rooted in the rejection of older forms of thinking – specifically, the work of Aristotle. But he does this in order to re-imagine how communities can be seen as developmental, teleological grounds of shared practice: much in the way that McBeath and Webb argue for an approach to social work that deepens its 'virtuous capacities' in order to increase workers' skills at analysing 'the shifting sands of cases, seeing them in a genuine ecological perspective instead of merely uttering, mantra-like, the word "ecological"' (2002: 1034).

The need to re-imagine community raises the first problem with MacIntyre's argument, from the perspective of social work. Throughout most of the world, it is the ideology of neoliberalism which underscores the resources (both materially and conceptually) for work with and within 'the community'. Governmental approaches are frequently shaped by their relation to wider economic policies at both a national and global level. For example, the 'personalisation' agenda within the UK arose in part from the disability rights movement (Glasby and Littlechild 2009); yet when articulated as government policy, successive regimes show 'less emphasis on the wider, emancipatory aspects of personalisation, as the focus tightens to a more reactive, individualistic perspective' (Lymbery 2012: 786). It seems, then, that while MacIntyre emphasises *practice* as the fundamental core of his vision of community, it is precisely at the *practical* level – and not the philosophical – that the 'ghostly' liberal self is most apparent.

Consider, for example, the 'Third Way' guiding New Labour policies, following their election to UK government in 1997, which were heavily influenced by the political communitarianism of Amitai Etzioni (1995). This aimed to steer between policies which led to rampant individualism (and thus inequality), and policies which created problems of welfare dependency (and thus increased taxation). Key to the 'Third Way' was an imperative that community be more than an 'abstract slogan': '"Community" doesn't imply trying to capture lost forms of local solidarity; it refers to practical means of furthering the social and material refurbishment of neighbourhoods, towns and larger local areas' (Giddens, 1998: 79). However, in practice the refusal of such policies to think outside of the neoliberal discourse that privileged the individual as a consumer first, and a relational actor second, ultimately undermined many of these initiatives, at least in the eyes of practitioners (Jordan and Jordan 2001; Pollock 2004; for a global comparative view, see Sen 2001). The result was that a renewed positive emphasis on community-focused projects such as Sure Start and the Social Exclusion Unit coincided with an opposing approach that continued to focus on individual assessment and 'casework'. Perhaps it is for this reason that MacIntyre has been insistent that his philosophy is *moral*, not political (see MacIntyre 1991).

This leads to a second question for communitarianism. If the ghostly individualism of the liberal arises in part from societal pluralism, then how do we decide *whose* shared identity, whose tradition and whose practices we should look to? Often, the examples of community held up by communitarians are rather too simplistic to be believable (Phillips 1993). Price and Simpson note that in moves towards community care for both service users with mental ill health, and those with learning disabilities, 'community is seen as some kind of ideal, a world in which neighbours care for each other, and where families support their own' (2007: 135); but that this is, in reality, a 'lost ideal' (136). They cite the charity Turning Point's (2004) highlighting of how, in the specific case of people with learning disabilities, integration into the community remains dependent on an idealised notion of 'caring neighbours', whilst neglecting material problems such as poor public services and real poverty. The communitarian examples of strong communities are often made so, not by the communal relations which bind them, but rather the power and privilege which allow their participants entry. But such power relations can very easily be obscured if, as the communitarian seems to suggest, the individual has no authority to challenge the community itself.

On this note, liberal philosophers such as Rawls have contested the caricaturing of their position as too 'abstract'. While they still value social interdependence (see Rawls 1996) they maintain certain rights must be preserved in order to be able to challenge any wrongdoing or oppression from within a community itself. Sometimes, these rights *have* to be abstract or assumed, rather than situated within communal virtues, in order to allow the experiences of the disadvantaged or excluded to be properly heard. Simon Duffy (2010), for example, engages with this kind of approach with his 'Citizenship Theory' regarding the valuing of the experiences of people with learning disabilities. From a slightly different perspective, Susan Moller Okin argues that because the experience of injustice is often deeply internalised or rationalised precisely through familial, communal and cultural relationships, the true nature of injustice may be concealed by the effects of socialisation. Thus, 'justice' cannot be decided simply by the members of a community. Instead, Okin claims that the *critical distance* of Rawls' original position is fundamental for the recognition of justice. This 'does not have to bring with it detachment; committed outsiders can often be better analysts and critics of social injustice than those who live within the relevant culture' (1998: 431).

Thinking through Practice

Asserting a rights-based, formalistic account of a community tends to emphasise individual freedom and choice; asserting a relational, genealogical account self necessarily highlights the communal traditions which form this. Kornbeck notes that while paying attention to situated communities helps to identify the lack of freedom of choice available to certain groups, this can risk 'over-ethnicising social problems and, worse, rejecting [...] aspirations for citizenship' of minority or under-represented groups (2001: 259).

How significant is this risk in your own practice or experience? Is it better, do you think, to approach the problem of community from a situated (e.g. communitarian) perspective, or a detached one (e.g. liberalist)?

Jean-Luc Nancy and the inoperative community

At first sight, the debate between liberal and communitarian viewpoints seems to cover the two basic positions available: we either see communities made of a group of individuals, or individuals as at least partially made up from the community around and within them. While Rawls recognises full well that individuals are embedded within complex relationships, he maintains that this should not affect the principle of justice. Communitarians are well aware that not all traditions are positive, and that tradition is a cause for marginalisation and oppression as well as formative moral support; but they see no other source of morality that would give justice meaning in reality. But because this can lead us into seemingly endless circles of debate, we may feel that somewhere the question of community has been missed once again. In which case, it may need to be looked at from another angle.

Such an angle has been offered by the work of Jean-Luc Nancy. Nancy does not offer any kind of 'third paradigm' between the two, though; his work is nuanced and complex, and does not benefit from the kind of summary we have space for here. What can be said, however, is that his work can be read as part of the debate on 'post-foundational' communities, alongside thinkers such as Alain Badiou, Jacques Rancière and Claude Lefort. Such thinkers all begin from the idea that any foundational principle of community can no longer be sustained or depended upon; if, indeed, it ever was. The problem with both liberalism and communitarianism, Nancy suggests, is that by reducing community to either principle – which both propose an account of community that is self-contained and undivided – we in fact undermine the basic sense of communal together-ness that relates people to each other in the first place. Instead, they lapse into a kind of 'totalitarianism': the domination of one idea of what the task or aim of community is.

He cites two particular characteristics of how the idea of community is employed today: 'communion' and 'work' (1991: 3). On the one hand, community can be fused together in the form of one figure: one social body, one activity, one leader and so on, which is similarly manufactured to operate according to a totalising view of what community is. This is a 'communion' – something Nancy identifies in 'actual existing communism' (1991: 3). In this case, the 'being-together' of community becomes a 'being *of* togetherness', and members of a community become de-individuated: think, for example, of the way in which ethnic minorities are frequently given a single persona as, for example, 'the Bangladeshi community' or 'the Irish Traveller community'.

On the other hand, the idea of community is invoked as something that needs to 'work': in other words it is something to be managed, operationalised, and organised. It is a functional, apolitical design based on the situating of buildings, workforces, populations and so on in order to ensure that a 'community' exists. While Nancy refers here to large-scale conceptions of work – perhaps something along the lines of Talcott Parson's functionalist sociology, or even Hayek's economic rationality – it can also be seen in more localised settings. Verity and Jolley (2008) discuss, for example, the sense in which a 'work-based' community is formed around an automative plant in Adelaide.

Here, the researchers found that definitive social bonds of community were formed by the shared cultural connections, kinship, shift organisation and the interdependence of the production process itself. It was only when the plant was closed down due to retrenchment, that the 'holistic view of the workplace in terms of the value of work-based social relations' became apparent by virtue of its loss (2008: 340).

> **Thinking through Practice**
>
> Earlier, you thought about how you defined the community you practised or worked within. Does either of Nancy's characteristics resonate with the definitions you gave?

Verity and Jolley's work echoes Nancy's point that the ways in which communities are *produced* from specifically political motivations can be hidden. Presuming that community is something that is simply 'there', self-identical and self-enclosed – which Nancy terms 'immanent' – leads to the view of community as something which emerges either organically, or from necessity. But it is, in fact, the very attempt to identify community as a 'characteristic' or principle which leads, inevitably, to the tensions and contradictions outlined at the start of the chapter: not least, the complex relationship between political agendas and funding guidelines aiming to use community to some end or purpose, and the experiences of those who live within spaces demarcated for such a 'community' that struggles to appear in as coherent and neat a way as politics demands. For this reason, philosophers come to depend upon some kind of 'original' community that has come before (Nancy 1991: 9): for Rawls, the original position, for MacIntyre, the pre-modern communities of Aristotle. But the fact that the history of philosophy has *always* shown a yearning for a lost, original community suggests that we should be suspicious of it referencing any specific or real community that once historically existed (1991: 10). Rather, we should see this as something constitutive of any attempt to formalise what community is. Paradoxically, the 'missing' of community is something inherent to community itself.

Thus Nancy turns the three ways of thinking through community we began with – thought, temporality and task – on their heads. For Nancy, the sense of being-in-common that philosophies of community search for, but inevitably overlook – what he terms our 'ontological sociality' (1991: 75) – *resists*, on an everyday level, the kind of tidy and reductive representations of community that both liberalism and communitarianism provide. This is because 'we are always in-common even before a being-communal can come into being' which 'deconstructs a priori every enclosing totality into which the individual would be absolved' (Devisch 2013: 107). Our shared existence is, paradoxically, radically other to the idea of a 'working' or 'communing' community itself. This aspect of our existence should be understood, not in terms of 'work' or 'communion', but rather as fundamentally 'inoperative'.

It should be apparent from his criticisms of liberalism and communitarianism that a simple and clear-cut statement of what he means by this will not do. It also means that his work can appear tortuously abstract, in order to avoid asserting any totalising view of what community should be. Nevertheless, we can outline two lines of thought that Nancy uses to support this claim: first, his critique of the 'retreat of the political' from contemporary thinking about the meaning of community; and second, his understanding of the 'ontological sociality' that gives people a 'being-in-common' at the level of practice.

The retreat of the political and the management of politics

Nancy distinguishes between 'politics' and the 'political' (in the French, this difference is marked by *le politique* and *la politique*). The former refers to the 'partisan strategies and concrete institutional devices' (Dallmayr 1997: 182), whereas the latter refers to the framework that these sit within, or that they presuppose in order to work. The 'political' is a kind of essence or authority of politics. It is, effectively, what replaces the older fixed order of authority within pre-modern feudal societies, where the figure of the King (or total ruler) was the centre of all power. Once that position is done away with in modern times, 'the political' is the space that replaces it. 'Politics', meanwhile, is the contestation for power *within* that space. The somewhat confusing similarity between the terms is, in fact, part of the point which Nancy wants to raise. He is concerned that the notion that seeing 'everything is politics' – as the radical social workers of the 1970s would claim – leads to a disappearance of, or 'retreat' from, the *political*. The utter obviousness that everything is political in some shape or form means that the *specificity* of what the political is becomes lost: such that if '*everything* is political, then *nothing* is anymore' (Nancy 2008: 25, my emphasis). Politics without the political is, Nancy argues, identical to having a society without community: it is simply a discussion of the ways in which people can be separated, disassociated and divided according to more abstract and ideal concepts and signs, without seeing the more fundamental 'communing' which this acts *upon* (1991: 11). It is thus 'society', not 'community', which Rawls and MacIntyre have been debating.

This is seen most clearly in Rawls's liberalist approach. His account of justice is rooted in a 'governing consensus' between the pluralism of 'reasonable comprehensive doctrines' (1996: 61). This, of course, means that such doctrines must have already accepted the basic tenets of liberalism in order to reach any consensus; otherwise, they are being unreasonable. This is clearly a political decision, but one which is curiously obscured in Rawls's own account. As Devisch argues:

> On the one hand, Rawls gives the impression that the period for philosophical debate and inquiry into *the political* is over and that *politics* is now first and foremost a problem of management, a kind of exercise for legal experts. […] On the other hand […] the choice to conceive of politics as the managing of a rational consensus capable of tolerating diversity is and remains a political choice, even if it presents itself as a postpolitical question. (2013: 153)

The problem of 'post-politics' speaks to the unspoken acceptance of particular forms of political structures. In turn, politics becomes a question of how to best carry out the authority of the political. Examples of this concern can be found throughout social work literature, chiefly regarding the dominance of neoliberal frameworks in the delivery of social care. For example, Donna Baines' study of social service restructuring in Canada argues that such a 'post-political' model has produced a 'narrowing of alternative visions of human service provision' (2006: 27); and while 'themes of worker "empowerment" reverberate through the private sector-like models of work organisation currently in vogue, workers' involvement with managerial processes rarely extends beyond new ways to streamline services, speed up delivery and meet workplace "performance goals"' (2006: 21). Hence, the 'politics' of social work became a matter of best procedure rather than radical change. Gray and Webb, meanwhile, critique the recent *Global Agenda for Social Work and Social Development* as being 'characteristic of a deepening process of de-politicization marked by the increasing evacuation of the proper political dimension from the public terrain as technocratic management and consensual policy-making sutures the spaces of democratic politics' (Gray and Webb 2014: 353–4).

For Nancy, this arises because we consider 'the social' only on its own terms; it has no reference beyond it to ground its existence, as we have no broader sense of 'the political' to authorise the arrangement of society (other than, perhaps: 'it seems to work'). Hence, the oft-cited phrase that originated with Fredric Jameson, and was used more recently by Mark Fisher (2009), that it is easier to imagine the end of the world than the end of capitalism. The reason – at least, according to Nancy – is that a society organised around the principle of operation (e.g. the free market) will simply refer to authority already within itself. The logic is circular. Nancy thus calls the bluff on Rawls and Okin's earlier appeal to the 'unencumbered self' as a way of 'thinking outside' particular community values: this still upholds an unspoken political ground based on its assumptions of how individuals reason with and relate to one another.

So what *is* the community?

Community, then, must mean something more integral about the *actual* relations between people – in Nancy's words, their 'being-in-common'. But at the same time we must resist the urge to 'represent' this as some kind of *principle* through which people are brought together. At its core, Nancy argues that 'community means, consequently, that there is no singular being without another singular being', which suggests 'an originary or ontological "sociality" that in principle extends far beyond the simple theme of man as a social being' (1991: 27).

Nancy's move towards an ontology of sociality seems very much in line with the approaches taken by the likes of Baines or Gray and Webb, when it articulates the need for resistance to this post-political order. But there does not exist, for Nancy, some kind of true community which lies before, behind or beyond the current arrangements of communities that we see today in, for example, the 'Islamic community', the 'learning disability community', and so on. As such, Nancy's response is almost deliberately frustrating, as he is keen to advocate any 'new' politics, or to simply substitute a community of 'work' with one of 'communion' based on the strength of shared cause or identity.

If his ontological sociality emphasises the significance of our everyday experiences of being-together, it also depends on recognising the vulnerability of such experiences, and their inherent resistance to any 'social bonds'. This reveals the paradoxical nature of community: that it is an exposure to our dependence on others; an exposure which itself allows us to be 'singular':

> A singular being *appears*, as finitude itself: at the end (or at the beginning), with the contact of the skin (or the heart) of another singular being, at the confines of the *same* singularity that is, as such, always *other*, always shared, always exposed. (1991: 27–8)

This sense of 'sharing' is not the same as MacIntyre's idea about shared practices and goals, however. As much as it is defined by its positive relations between people, Nancy sees community as an *ending* of relations with other people: communities come into being when borders between the in-group and out-group are drawn; just as my sense of being a singular being arises from my awareness of separation from another. Sharing, Nancy suggests, 'comes down to this: what community reveals to me [...] is my existence outside myself. [...] *Community itself, in sum, is nothing but this exposition*. It is the community of finite beings, and as such it is itself a *finite* community' (1991: 26–7).

Of course, Nancy is not offering some kind of psychosocial theory here; rather, he is deconstructing the more conventional accounts of how we 'miss' community in order to show the paradoxical way in which community is recognised. Community is 'formed by the retreat or by the subtraction of something [...]. [I]t is the work that the community does *not* do and that it *is* not that forms community' (Nancy 1991: xxxix). It is from *this* perspective that Nancy mourns the loss of community. Not, as Tönnies argued, as a nostalgic loss of something which once existed before (i.e. the community is replaced by society; intimate relations are replaced by economically-driven and abstract divisions), or as the work of MacIntyre suggests (i.e. that community needs to be realised in order for the world to allow the atomistic, individualistic modern society make sense). Both assume the contours of what a community 'is', and proceed from this. Nancy, meanwhile, highlights the loss of an *awareness* of the ontological basis upon which the *meaning* of community is structured. In Devisch's words, it is 'not that people cannot feel connected to each other, it is rather that this connectedness is momentary and never total in itself'. So, while group identity and culture exists – there are, of course, Islamic communities, learning disabilities movements, and so on – 'these identities are always internally divided. [...] Identities never simply coincide with themselves, but always form and reform anew' (Devisch 2013: 107). The social bonds that produce such representations of community 'only [exist] insofar as [they] must be continuously retied' (108).

Ironically, perhaps, Nancy's appeal for establishing the inoperativeness of community is 'everydayness'. The elusiveness of his writing can conceal the fact that this being-in-common is not abstract, but lived, situated and localised. It is by realising that our sense of being-in-common with others on the ground is as affective and constitutive of our sense of community as any sense of work or communal affiliation – the ways we encounter a voice of a service user at the end of the phone, whom you will never meet; or an image of a child in the news that stirs a response; or the touch of a loved one on your return from work – that allows us to challenge either the nostalgic yearnings of communitarianism, or the post-political inevitability of liberalism. It does so by problematising the 'safe opposition between intimate encounters with our "own" people and anonymous contact with far-off strangers' (Devisch 2013: 116) that conventional, self-enclosed accounts of community provide. This is not proposing some kind of glib sense of universal humanity; this would be simply another claim to '*the* truth of the community', and a further retreat from 'the political'. Rather, they show how our everyday encounters – a 'sharing' built not on rights, property or goals, but rather on the sense that what we share is *also* what divides us; our identity-with is *also* a difference-from; hence such 'places of communication' are 'defined and exposed by their dislocation' (Nancy 1991: 25) – puncture any totalising communal identity, however positive or negative this may be.

Thinking through Practice

Donna Baines notes that:

> The commitment of social work to provide voice and self-determination to clients [...] finds compatibility with community experiments aimed at inverting power structures so that those previously silenced within institutional agendas are provided with voice, resources and collective power. (2006: 30)

The work of Nancy is an exploration of the question of community that refuses to defend any 'model' or 'theory' of community itself. How important might such an exploration be, do you think, for planning and promoting such 'community experiments'?

Notes

1 The word 'liberal' – no less than the word 'community' – has a number of different, and often conflicting meanings. In this case, it is being used in the sense of modern political philosophy: that is, the pursuit of criteria for judging rationality and morality independent from tradition or context, with an emphasis on fairness, toleration and procedural, rather than teleological, governance.

2 McBeath and Webb note that while there were some attempts within the 1980s to directly engage social work ethics and MacIntyre's revival of 'virtue-based' communitarianism, these 'fell stillborn from the presses' (2002: 1019).

References

Anderson, B. (1983). *Imagined Communities*. London: Verso.
Ayre, P. (2007). 'Common Ground'. *Community Care*, No. 1666, pp. 36–7.
Baines, D. (2006) 'Social Work and Neo-liberalism: "If You Could Change One Thing": Social Service Workers and Restructuring.' *Australian Social Work*, 59, 1, 20–34.
Brown, W. (2005). *Edgework: Critical Essays on Knowledge and Politics*. Princeton, NJ: Princeton University Press.
Dallmayr, F. (1997). 'An "Inoperative" Global Community? Reflections on Nancy.' In Sheppard, D., Sparks, S. and Thomas, C. (eds.), *On Jean-Luc Nancy: The Sense of Community*. London: Routledge, pp. 174–96.
Devisch, I. (2013). *Jean-Luc Nancy and the Question of Community*. London: Bloomsbury.
Dominelli, L. (2004). *Social Work: Theory and Practice for a Changing Profession*. Cambridge: Polity Press.
Duffy, S. (2010). 'The Citizenship Theory of Social Justice: Exploring the Meaning of Personalisation for Social Workers.' *Journal of Social Work Practice*, 24, 3, 253–67.
Dworkin, R. (1981). 'What is Equality? Part 1: Equality of Welfare.' *Philosophy and Public Affairs*, Vol. 10, pp. 185–246.
Etzioni, A. (1995). *The Spirit of Community: Rights, Responsibilities, and the Communitarian Agenda*. London: Fontana.
Featherstone, M. (1995). *Undoing Culture: Globalisation, Postmodernism and Identity*. London: Sage.
Fisher, M. (2009). *Capitalist Realism: Is There No Alternative?* London: Zero Books.
Fynsk, C. (1991). 'Foreword: Experiences of Finitude.' In Nancy, J. (ed.), *The Inoperative Community*. Minneapolis, MN: Minnesota University Press, pp. vii–xxxv.
Garland, D. (2001). *The Culture of Control*. Oxford: Oxford University Press.
Garrett, P. (2013). *Social Work and Social Theory*. Bristol: Policy Press.
Giddens, A. (1998). *The Third Way*. Cambridge: Polity Press.
Glasby, J. and Littlechild, R. (2009). *Direct Payments and Personal Budgets: Putting Personalisation into Practice*. Bristol: Policy Press.
Gray, M. and Webb, S. (2014). 'The Making of a Civil Society Politics in Social Work: Myth and Misrepresentation with the Global Agenda.' *International Social Work*, 57, 4, 346–59.
Groys, B. (2010). *Going Public*. New York: Steinberg Press.
Held, V. (1999). 'Feminist Transformations of Moral Theory.' In Sterba, J. (ed.), *Ethics: The Big Questions*. Oxford: Blackwell, pp. 331–45.
Hobbes, T. (1972 [1651]). *De Homine and De Cive [Man and Citizen]*. Garden City, NY: Doubleday and Company.
Hopkins, P. and Hill, M. (2010). 'The Needs and Strengths of Unaccompanied Asylum-Seeking Children and Young People in Scotland.' *Child and Family Social Work*, 15, 4, 399–408.
Jordan, B. and Jordan, C. (2001). *Social Work and the Third Way: Tough Love as Social Policy*. London: Sage.
Keay, D. (1987) 'Interview for *Woman's Own*.' Available online at: http://www.margaretthatcher.org/document/106689

Koeske, G. F., Lichtenwalter, S. and Koeske, R. D. (2005). 'Social Workers' Current and Desired Involvement in Various Practice Activities: Exploration and Implications.' *Administration in Social Work*, 29, 2, 63–83.

Kornbeck, J. (2001). '"Gemeinschaft" skills versus "Gesellschaft" Skills in Social Work Education and Practice: Applying Tönnies' Dichotomy for a Model of Intercultural Communication.' *Social Work Education*, 20, 2, 247–61.

Lane, M. (1999). 'Community Development and a Postmodernism of Resistance.' In Fook, J. and Pease, B. (eds), *Transforming Social Work Practice: Postmodern Critical Perspectives*. London: Routledge, pp. 135–49.

Lewis, J. A., Lewis, M. D., Packard, T. and Souflee, F. (2001). *Management of Human Service Programs*. 3rd edn. Belmont, CA: Brooks/Cole.

Levi-Strauss, C. (1981). *Introduction to a Science of Mythology 4: The Naked Man*. New York: Harper & Row.

Lymbery, M. (2005). *Social Work with Older People*. London: Sage.

—— (2012). 'Social Work and Personalisation.' *British Journal of Social Work*, 42, 783–92.

Lynn, M. (2006). 'Discourses of Community: Challenges for Social Work.' *International Journal of Social Welfare*, 15, 110–20.

McBeath, G. and Webb, S. (2002). 'Virtue, Ethics and Social Work: Being Lucky, Realistic and Not Doing One's Duty.' *British Journal of Social Work*, 32, 1015–36.

MacIntyre, A. (1981). *After Virtue*. London: Gerald Duckworth and Co. Ltd.

—— (1991). 'I'm Not a Communitarian, But…' *The Responsive Community*, 1, 3, 91–2.

Maslow, A. (1970) *Motivation and Personality*. London: Harper and Row.

Nancy, J. (1991). *The Inoperative Community*, P. Connor, L. Garbus, M. Holland, and S. Sawhney (trans.). Minneapolis, MN: Minnesota University Press.

Nozick, R. (1974). *Anarchy, State and Utopia*. New York: Basic Books.

Okin, S. M. (1998). 'Gender Inequality and Cultural Difference.' In Sterba, J. (ed.), *Ethics: The Big Questions*. Oxford: Blackwell, pp. 422–34.

Pavelová, L. (2014). 'Community Work or Community Social Work?', *Revista de Asistență Socială*, 13, 1, 7–15.

Phillips, D. (1993). *Looking Backward: A Critical Appraisal of Communitarian Thought*. Princeton, NJ: Princeton University Press.

Pollock, A. (2004). *NHS, PLC: the Privatisation of our Health Care*. London: Verso.

Powell, F. and Geoghegan, M. (2004). *The Politics of Community Development*. Dublin: A & A Farmar.

Price, V. and Simpson, G. (2007). *Transforming Society? Social Work and Sociology*. Bristol: Policy Press.

Rawls, J. (1971). *A Theory of Justice*. Cambridge, MA: Harvard University Press.

—— (1996). *Political Liberalism*. New York: Columbia University Press.

Rose, N. (1996). 'The Death of the Social? Re-figuring the Territory of Government.' *Economy and Society*, 25, 3, 327–56.

Rothman, C.J. (2008). *Cultural Competence in Process and Practice: Building Bridges*. Boston, MA: Allyn & Bacon.

Schirmer, W. and Michailakis, D. (2015). 'The Lost *Gemeinschaft*: How People Working with the Elderly Explain Loneliness.' *Journal of Aging Studies*, 33, 1–10.

Sen, K. (ed.) (2001). *Restructuring Health Services: Changing Contexts and Comparative Perspectives*. London: Zed Books.

Tönnies, F. (2003). *Community and Society*. London: Dover Publications.

Turning Point (2004). *Hidden Lives*. London: Turning Point.

Verity, F. and Jolley, G. (2008). 'Closure of an Automotive Plant: Transformation of a Work-based "Community".' *Policy Studies*, 29, 3, 331–41.

Ward, G. (2005). *Cultural Transformation and Religious Practice*. Cambridge: Cambridge University Press.

Webb, S. (2006). *Social Work in a Risk Society*. Basingstoke: Palgrave Macmillan.

Wilkinson, R. (2005). *The Impact of Inequality: How to Make Sick Societies Healthier*. London: Routledge.

Zimbardo, P. (1971). 'The Power and Pathology of Imprisonment.' Congressional Record (Serial No. 15, 1971-10-25). Washington, DC: US Government Printing Office.

3
IDENTITY

A short word from Nietzsche: marginalisation, recognition and *ressentiment*

The problem with valuing people

In 2001 the UK Department of Health introduced the *Valuing People* policy. A key part of the 'personalisation' agenda, the policy aimed to promote social inclusion for people with learning disabilities, continuing the long-term move away from state-controlled institutional care, and towards a quasi-market of consumer choice and service user 'control'. This was shaped, according to Vicky Price and Graeme Simpson, by a 'triumvirate' of influences: 'liberal economics; liberal, or potentially radical, social work and social welfare opinion; and the crucial element of service user led movements, who located themselves outside of Government agencies in the struggle for social justice' (2009: 182). Despite arising from different interests, ideologies and histories, these three influences all share, on the surface at least, a commitment to some form of 'liberation' from centralised monopolies – whether this is a monopoly on what is 'right' or 'appropriate' care for a service user to receive, or what should or should not be invested in.

However, Price and Simpson go on to bring attention to four case studies, based on empirical practice examples, that 'show how the drive towards supported or community based provision can result in greater levels of vulnerability' (2009: 184). Their focus on the lived experience of service users allows them to further highlight Burton and Kagan's (2006) critique of the policy as being overly shaped by neo-liberal agendas over and above that of service user led social change. They point to a lack of value in care provision itself beyond its economic costings (Price and Simpson 2009: 183); the expectations of familial and community support for service users; and the imbalance between the speed with which institutional care is withdrawn compared to the amount and range of medium-and long-term support provision (185). 'Perhaps,' they suggest, 'the greater indictment is the paradoxical levels of isolation and exclusion the implementation brought about' (184).

Such a policy is certainly not alone in producing a paradox between the aspirations of inclusion leading, in certain cases, to the further exclusion and disempowering of those on the margins. There is no need to recount here the immense amount of work that has been done on anti-oppressive practice, anti-discriminatory practice, service user discourses, survivor narratives, and so on, that both highlight and respond to this problem of exclusion. That social work involves allowing previously silenced voices to be heard is central to the ethos of practice (Cree and Davis 2006; Dalrymple and Burke 1995). For Lena Dominelli, social work's core values involve articulating and advocating service user perspectives on the basis of 'citizenship', which allows social workers to critically identify 'the gap between theoretical and actual citizenship' (Dominelli 2004: 232); just as Price and Simpson use it to identify the gap between the potential benefits of *Valuing People* and its inherent risks.

But while it goes almost without saying that social work knowledge must attend to the service user perspective, the risk remains that appeals to 'lived experience' become platitudinous rather than effective. As Potts and Brown dryly remark, given the choice between being oppressive or anti-oppressive, 'hopefully we would all choose the latter' (2008: 50); but the rhetoric of such a norm can often suggest two clearly defined 'sides' when the reality may well be more complex. Writing in a different context, the Nietzsche scholar James Hans has noted how easily the distinction between the hegemonic voices on the 'inside', and the lived experience on the 'outside', can slip into facile value distinctions of what is 'good' and what is 'bad'. Such a value distinction echoes the paradox regarding the effects of inclusion: 'Under the banners of "openness" and "tolerance" and "non-difference" and the like, one tends to find only a different kind of closedness, intolerance and redifferentiation' (Hans 1992: 15). A simplistic division between the authenticity of the margins and the hegemony of the centre is problematic, though. Writing in the context of mental health services, Crossley and Crossley alert us to the problems that the *speed* of such a judgement might bring:

> 'Listen to the voice of the user!' 'Let survivors and consumers speak out!' Such sentiments are commonplace within the contemporary mental health field, even if many pay no more than lip service to them. [...] But what is this 'voice'? Is it, as the more 'existential' passages in Foucault's *Madness and Civilisation* might lead us to believe, the ahistorical 'other' of contemporary forms of medical power; a subjugated but authentic discourse which might be recovered and restored through progressive political measures? Or is it, like the voice of medicine, a constructed voice; a historical invention? (Crossley and Crossley 2001: 1477)

Thinking through Practice

How would you respond to Crossley and Crossley's question? Are there alternative routes to an answer than 'historical invention' or 'ahistorical "other"'?

This problem resonates not only within social work theory but also in philosophical discussions on gender, disability, race, and other forms of significant difference. *From where* does marginalised identity speak? How is it *produced*? How is it *listened* to? How does it *critique* existing traditions of knowledge, power and social care? If critiques of exclusionary policies such as Price and Simpson's are to be fully effective, these are questions which need to be answered, given that they depend upon us taking seriously the views of service users who are engaged in the personalisation agenda.

I will not, however, attempt to answer these questions here. This chapter is instead, as advertised, a short word from the nineteenth century German philosopher Friedrich Nietzsche. Nietzsche may seem an odd interlocutor, given how rarely he appears in social work textbooks; and perhaps for obvious reasons, given his fiercely anti-egalitarian views, his arguments against the value of 'compassion' and 'the task of the healthy to nurse the sick' (1997: 92), and that his name frequently conjures images of a misogynist forerunner to Nazism. The caricatures of Nietzsche's thought can hide the complexity of both his philosophy and his writing, but the significance of his critique of the ideas of truth and morality in western philosophy remains. If one problem of allowing silenced voices to be heard is how we separate platitude from effective practice, then responding to such radical voices is one way to articulate this.

Some paradoxes of inclusion

The problem of inclusion – whether political, social, epistemological or philosophical – often circulates around whether 'inclusion' entails a right of the marginalised to be 'equal' with those who are not marginalised, or a right to be 'different', and have this difference recognised as significant and valuable, rather than deficient. In other words, it is a question of whether inclusion amounts to *assimilation* or *differentiation*. If inclusion is a case of assimilation, then we must be confident that the governing values of equality are fit to accommodate marginalised perspectives. This is broadly in line with Dominelli's view of 'citizenship': that while some voices are silenced, this is because the values of citizenship are not being upheld consistently. By advocating for service users, social workers can effectively hold society more accountable to its principles of equality. This also reflects the liberal humanism of Rawls or Habermas: inclusion is a procedural issue.

Conversely, the idea of inclusion as differentiation refuses to pretend that such equality can exist, and that a 'one size fits all' approach will not attend to the specific problems faced by those who have been marginalised or disempowered. This is because the apparent 'equality' of existing systems of representation can be argued to themselves be representative of specific, privileged viewpoints – typically male, typically white, typically higher class (see Harding 1991). In this sense, the 'service user voice' is not simply wanting to be heard *alongside* those of the social worker, the local authority, or the general public, etc., but rather to be heard in terms of the unique perspective they bring which would otherwise not be recognised. In doing so, the aim is to lessen the power of the centralised voices in discussions and decision-making processes, rather than to simply join their ranks. But this, in turn, gives rise to what is often termed the 'difference dilemma': in revaluing the significance of a service user perspective, the risk is to essentialise that perspective. In short: 'how is it possible to identify and provide services to a group without, at the same time, labelling and stigmatising that group?' (Parker *et al.* 1999: 151).

These two views on inclusion are, of course, archetypal, and the route towards including the 'service user voice' rarely follows one path or the other exclusively. This is in part due to the complex nature of how the 'service user voice' is hermeneutically *produced*. The very notion of a 'service user voice' depends on identity categories which will already affect the way it is heard. Identity is invariably identification *with* something. As Connolly explains, 'an identity is established in relation to a series of differences that have become socially recognized. […] If they did not coexist as differences, it would not exist in its distinctness and solidity' (Connolly 2002: 64). In this way, marginal identities do not exist *separate* from the more centralised ones; rather, they sit on the 'edge' of our accepted, ready-to-hand models of identity, and are defined dialectically through these (Taylor 1995). Often, this renders the marginal only recognised as the opposite of the centre. While complete exclusion from a representative system (politics, social care, philosophy, etc.) would equate to a literal non-existence, more often marginalised subjects are 'seen' and 'heard' fairly constantly within mainstream discussions; but hermeneutically framed in terms of their disempowered status (see Le Doeuff 1989). Hence, Jenny Morris has criticised the term 'people with disabilities' because it defines them by impairment, and thus 'robs us of the language we need to describe oppression and discrimination' (Morris 2001: 3). Mental health service users, likewise, could be said to be highly *visible* within modern political debates, but only in terms of their 'dangerousness' or 'risk' (Beresford 2005: 33). It's not quite as simple, then, as dispelling stereotypes with appeals to 'real' people and 'real' voices. Our engagement with marginalised identities is always mediated; we come into contact with them for a reason, and through certain interpretative channels. For a subject to become politically effective, rather than caricatured 'other', then they must challenge the established framework for identification.

Thinking through Practice

Asking what the available images of personhood are for those diagnosed with dementia, Mitchell *et al.* note that popular literature – replete with book titles such as *Death in Slow Motion* or *The Living Dead: Alzheimer's in America* – is beset with a discourse of decaying monstrosity: 'These images, coupled as they usually are with the tragedy discourse of being doomed, gutted, ravaged, taken over by a beast, and turned into the living dead, perpetuate a deep and pernicious fear of, and disregard for, persons with dementia' (Mitchell *et al.*

2013: 2). Behuniak (2011) thus argues that the diagnosis of Alzheimer's being linked to the representation of dementia as 'the walking dead', is reflective of a broader cultural interest in zombies in the US.

To what extent do marginalised identities speak through the images of popular culture? How might this problematise the equality/difference debate? How, alternatively, might this shape the interpretative relationship between social worker and service user?

Appearances of inclusion

For Jacques Rancière, the question instead revolves around what he terms the 'distribution of the sensible': that is, 'the way in which the abstract and arbitrary forms of symbolization of hierarchy are embodied as perceptive givens, in which a social destination is anticipated by the evidence of a perceptive universe, of a way of being, saying and seeing' (2011: 7). For Rancière, at the heart of any politics there is an *aesthetic* dimension that orders what can be seen and talked about and what can't. The question of marginalised identity is, then, not one of tolerating different interest groups within a shared space of discussion, but rather a question of *how things appear* as images and voices, and whether these are meaningful or otherwise. And this is often why the equality/difference debate can fall short when it appeals to an essentialised or fixed sense of identity, whether expressed in terms of the reductive principles of equality, or the marks of difference. The 'lived experience' of a service user does not simply appear without any kind of interpretative framing; rather it often has a framing which bears resistance and struggle:

> Often we do not want to be seen as service users; not just because we are aware of the loss of status involved and possible disempowerment, but because of the ways in which our lives and identities may be remade to fit the identity of service user. Yet in order for 'good social work' to take place, there may be a need for people to fit the relevant identity categories. (Fook 2002: 78)

Putting the language of popular culture to one side, then, we can see that this interpretative framing is at work in more specific ways, in the concern for 'good social work'. There are further implications when we consider the relationship between 'identity' and the ways in which social care is given meaning within a late modern neoliberal context. As Thornton notes, while identity categories can be strategically useful, they lend themselves to a discourse of consumer rights which depends upon fixed and essentialist categories ('person with a disability', 'care leaver', 'ethnic minority'), over and above the more 'temporal and fluid' process of identity formation (Thornton 2000: 20). Hence, 'gaps' between theoretical and actual citizenship may emerge from listening to the service user voice, as Dominelli describes; but in doing so might also leave 'dominant meaning systems [...] unquestioned', resulting in cases where 'even subordinate groups act against their own self-interest, because they unwittingly comply with the dominant discourse' (Fook 2002: 66). In the case of *Valuing People*, this is embedded within the pervasive influence of neoliberalism within social policy (see Clarke 2004; Jones 2004) which promises equality in the form of consumer identity, but is accompanied by *depoliticising* narratives that 'make nearly everything seem a matter of individual agency or will, on the one hand, or fortune or contingency on the other' (Brown 2006: 18). Hence, in some cases rights-based approaches to social work may begin from a position of emancipation, but instead place the burden of change on to the individual rather than the social context surrounding them; or, to put it more bluntly, the individual is given rights *only* in order to take responsibility for being wrong.

In this sense, the problem cannot necessarily be resolved with distinctions such as Ferguson's (2008), between 'top-down' (a consumerist concern with 'involvement') and 'bottom-up' (an activist concern with social change) approaches to service user involvement in the construction of social work knowledge. The issue is instead the nature of the *antagonism* between marginalised voice and centralised knowledge. This is perhaps reflected in Crossley and Crossley's argument regarding the tone of 'demand' in service user discourses:

> The increasing sense of the validity of personal experiences leads to a new voice of demand. If what 'we' are saying is correct, if 'we' have all suffered oppression and depersonalisation at the hands of 'the professionals', then 'we' have a 'right', an 'entitlement' and an obligation to those of 'us' who have suffered silently, to push for our group's desires and demands. [...]
>
> It is this understanding of oppression as a collective, system-based phenomenon, which leads to an intrinsic sense of 'right' and 'entitlement'. If 'the system' cannot be trusted to treat 'us' in the manner 'we' deserve, then we have to 'fight' that system. (Crossley and Crossley 2001: 1485)

What Crossley and Crossley describe here sits uncomfortably between, on the one hand, the recognition that personal experience is not simply idiosyncratic and individualised, but rather reflective of the broader marginalisation of certain voices – in other words, the positive and constructive forms of service user led reform – and on the other hand what Žižek terms 'ultra-politics', whereby the very conflict that this raises is depoliticised by virtue of a foreclosed 'us' and 'them' (2011: 71). Interest groups and activist collectives necessarily depend upon determined identities. Healy notes how 'groups of individuals such as women, indigenous people and people with disabilities can be said to share certain experiences by virtue of their shared location', which are also 'classified by reference to various social categories, such as class, gender, race and ethnicity, disability and sexuality' (1999: 119). This works to the extent that shared and representable interests can be promoted and place their demands upon the political system (see Sapiro 1998). But it also risks mediating experience through a reductive lens.

The problem with this is twofold. First, as McLaughlin rightly notes, 'the idea of a service user, as a homogenised entity, is to reduce all of those who use services to be viewed through the prism of one aspect of their lives' (2012: 136). To represent an identity as marginalised is to already re-frame the appearance of the individual in terms of particular needs or exclusion. Second, this grounds the engagement between marginalised and centralised identities as one of representative interest, *rather* than the kind of 'lived experience' that Price and Simpson reported in their critique of *Valuing People*. This second problem raises a further issue regarding the prevalence of the 'voice' as the primary form of expression – whether literal or metaphorical – and whether this privileges certain communicative forms over and above others. Indeed, highlighting the 'voice' or 'view' of the service user can conceal its relationship to the production of knowledge in terms of propriety and authorship: as Wilson and Beresford (2000) note, early attempts to bring service user voices to the centre of practice relied on institutional 'experts' (academics and service professionals) appropriating the experiences of service users in order to construct a theory, authored, ultimately, by the professionals themselves.

> **Thinking through Practice**
>
> Discussing some potential risks with the idea of 'activist social work', Karen Healy notes that 'regardless of the transformative strategies employed, the very presence of professional workers is disabling for service users'; and that, 'by virtue of their privilege, [social workers can] reproduce the oppression of service users' (1999: 120).
>
> To what extent might the power inherent in the professional role affect how one 'hears' the voices of service users? Think about your own practice, or understanding of the social work role. In what specific places, and through what specific acts and engagements, does the interpretative framing of such voices take place? For example, would you agree with McLaughlin (2007) that the very titles of 'client', 'service user', 'expert by experience' carry with them implications for how such a voice 'appears'?

Hanley *et al.* are critical of the notion that voices from the margins should be seen as representative of anything more than those singular experiences; and hence, for them, it is important to think 'about seeking perspectives rather than representativeness' (2004: 5), and that the range of perspectives contributes to a wider understanding of an issue. But while this seems to initially overcome the problem of essentialising service user 'interests', the reduction of social work knowledge to a collection of 'perspectives' has its own problems. Indeed, seeking individual 'perspectives' rather than a 'representation' of service user experience would seem to lead us back in a circle. For one's 'perspective' is not essential or natural (otherwise, wouldn't 'perspective' *equate* to 'representativeness'?), but rather emerges from, and is articulated through, a network of conditions and contexts that establish one's viewpoint or experience of a particular issue or identity. Indeed, Crossley and Crossley conclude their investigation into the service user voice in mental health contexts by arguing that 'the "voice" of users is structured by historically specific habits or habitus but those habits are, in turn, sediments of prior struggles from which they have emerged' (2001: 1489). The question, then, is not so much one of drawing a clear line between the authentic, individual view of one service user or other, and the socially and culturally determinant contexts that shape their discourse. Rather, the question is a more practical one: what do these differences between the production of a service user 'voice' mean in terms of where they take us forward to, critically and reflectively?

Nietzsche's challenge: *ressentiment* and reactive power

It is on this point – the fundamentally practical point regarding the relationship between service user voice and the 'sediments of prior struggles' – that we turn to the history of philosophy for our 'short word' from Nietzsche.[1] Nietzsche's work advocated a form of 'perspectivism' which asserted that there are no facts – of identity or experience – which speak for themselves. Thus, the 'perspectives' that Hanley *et al.* refer to are, for Nietzsche, always processes of interpretation, rather than an epistemological uncovering of a pre-existing meaning. Identifying a service user voice as such involves layers of production techniques – necessary, of course, for anything like 'social work knowledge' or 'policy critique' to emerge, but techniques nonetheless, which decipher the significance of what such perspectives 'mean' (Schrift 1990: 173). This does not make them any less 'real', but rather draws attention, again, to the interpretative framing that allows us to recognise them.

Within this interpretative context, Nietzsche suggests that the force of such perspectives can be seen in terms of their *action* and *reaction*. This corresponds to what Nietzsche, in a somewhat off-putting manner for contemporary readers, terms 'noble' and 'slave' morality. While the terms 'noble' and 'slave' may conjure images of medieval class warfare,[2] Nietzsche is rather attempting to account for why particular moral values have become prevalent within European society, when they seem to result in confused and contradictory tensions; precisely the kind of tensions we see in our question over what is valued about the service user voice, and what is not. For Nietzsche, values are always inherently political, and reflect the interests of those who utilise the most effective forms of power. But crucially – and controversially – for Nietzsche, such power is held by the 'slave', rather than the 'noble' (Nietzsche 1997: 50–2). While the 'active force' of the noble dominates, and 'reactive force' is dominated, reactive force is still powerful. In subordinating oneself to the dominant order, and to adapt to the existing principles of society, one is still expressing a force: 'Illness, for example, separates me from what I can do, as reactive force it makes me reactive, it narrows my possibilities and condemns me to a diminished milieu to which I can do no more than adapt myself' (Deleuze 2006: 61). This force that allows adaptation is nevertheless a force: 'it endows me with a new will that I can make my own' (61), albeit a will predicated only on my own dissatisfaction.

Reactive forces become conscious in human beings in the form of *ressentiment*. This French term is not to be confused with 'resentment'; although the two can blur. Resentment, as a moral and political concept, arises from the liberal tradition of thought; most notably the liberal economist Adam Smith, who in the eighteenth century wrote that it was a 'disagreeable' but nevertheless necessary aspect of social existence. Resentment arises as a reaction to the pain inflicted by another; and is directed, not towards the returning of pain, but rather towards making the perpetrator 'conscious that he feels it upon his past conduct, to make him repent of that conduct', and 'that the person whom he injured did not deserve to be treated in that manner' (Smith 1977: 94–7). Resentment is not vengeance, because it is tempered by the moral duties of society: which is, in the familiar liberal manner, determined by impartial and rational judgement on what is fair. In this sense we have a basic liberal construction of how marginalised voices can identify wrongs in a system. Resentment can thus be a key part of maintaining inclusivity, as it provides both a defence against wrongdoing (people notice when they are being treated badly), and in turn calls for its recognition and alleviation. This moral aspect is what distinguishes it from mere envy (Rawls 1971: 533). In doing so, the language of liberalism speaks to a simplistic division between justice and injustice, and inclusion and exclusion. If we have already agreed on the rules of engagement, then we simply allow every viewpoint the freedom to be expressed. In this sense, resentment is a passing act or emotion, which is framed by an ideal of equality: it arises when the agreed amount of respect is not being given.

Nietzsche questioned the basis of this ideal by applying a genealogical method to examine the origin of concepts, usually considered to be transcendent or universal – such as equality, difference, 'good' and 'evil', and so on – which underlie and structure our values. *Ressentiment* thus represents a longer-term feeling than resentment, as well as a fundamental failure for those wanting revenge to actually enact it. Because those who feel *ressentiment* are fundamentally weakened, they cannot simply respond in kind to those who marginalise them (it is worth noting, though, that while it is clear that Nietzsche's concept of 'slave morality' arises from those who feel *ressentiment* on the basis of structural or social disadvantage – gender, race, disability and so on – he utterly ignores any kind of economic basis for such categories emerging, even if their feeling of *ressentiment* was rooted within their lack of access to resources). Instead, they can enact symbolic or imaginary acts of revenge: which, for Nietzsche, manifests itself in the system of morality (1997: 20). Thus, the entire liberal paradigm of tolerance and inclusion is itself the product of a deep-rooted and frustrated sense of alienation and persecution. Inclusion *itself* is a reactive force.

Ressentiment and social theory

While the language of Nietzsche's account is largely a response to the culture of nineteenth century Europe, contemporary thinkers such as Slavoj Žižek have argued that such an account of *ressentiment* can be levelled at the forms of 'identity politics' and differentiation approaches to social inclusion. Karen Healy notes how such an approach can be liberating for service user movements 'when one comes to challenge negative stereotypes about the self as issues not of personal deficit but of structural oppression', but when this results in an insistence on 'victimhood', this can also 'limit one's capacity for power by placing responsibility for change in the hands of the other, more power person/group, and by limiting one's identity as the stigmatized self' (2005: 81). As Hoggett *et al.* note, while 'at first sight it might be thought there is little psychological or material advantage in being a victim', there are certain compensations that may well include 'a particular a sense of moral superiority with regard to the one towards whom one's complaints are directed' (2013: 6). On Nietzsche's account, then, we might say that while marginalised perspectives draw power from their identity *as* marginalised, this risks resulting in a reactive, rather than active, power. The marginalised groups thus identify with their own marginalisation as a source of strength; in turn, that which marginalises them becomes essential for channelling their blame.

In this way, marginalised identity becomes *both* politicised – in the sense of having a clear aim or 'other' that is the target of its critique: social services, care provision, the welfare budget, etc. – and simultaneously *depoliticised*, because such an 'other' is necessarily beyond harm. Thus, for Max Scheler, who developed a sociological account of the concept in the 1960s:

> Revenge [...] becomes transformed into *ressentiment* the more it is directed against lasting circumstances that are deemed injurious but beyond one's control. In some cases, the circumstances constitute an abstraction, such as 'the establishment,' 'the system,' 'the government,' or 'the economy' – all seen as especially invulnerable. (Meltzer and Musolf 2002: 244; see Scheler 1992: 116–143)

It should be added that this obviously works both ways. The affluent middle classes may identify abstractions of welfare recipients in much the same way: hence the 'visibility' we referred to previously of marginalised groups such as the long-term disabled and mental health service users. Insecurity and fear can be projected on to those who do not 'fit', or 'contribute', or drain resources. The 'transiency and suffering' which define the conditions of each perspective 'can be tolerated best if humans can find some agent who is responsible for suffering, an agent who can become the repository of resentment' (Connolly 1988: 153). And this, in many ways, reads as an alternative account to Crossley and Crossley's earlier narrative of how interest groups emerged, and forms the basis of Žižek's 'ultra-politics'.

As mentioned earlier, such reactive responses are not momentary or fleeting, but embedded within the 'sediments of prior struggles': that is, they are bred from what Gadamer would term the 'historically effected consciousness' (2004: 391) that forms our interpretative horizons (although Gadamer also notes that 'Nietzsche has more to say about the abuse than the use of history for life' (1999: 96)). In total contrast to the liberal notion of resentment, which focused on individual acts, *ressentiment* is not simply a psychological affect, but an interpretative organisation of lived experiences, communal histories and narratives, cultural myths and societal values. Healy suggests that a prime example of the application of this affective response to difference within social work practice arises within the discourse of 'consumer rights' as a vehicle for service user voices. Configuring service user groups in terms of 'consumer' identities has often proved useful in helping both to challenge accepted divisions between 'normal' and 'abnormal', and highlight the structural deficiencies that create them. However, fuelled by the historical narrative of exclusion, Healy suggests that:

> in some contexts, consumer rights discourse goes beyond a critique of powerful health and welfare institutions to criticise the power wielded by professionals. In this interpretation, professional service providers are caricatured as self-interested and oppressive [...] preventing us from recognising the difference within the powerful group from using these to achieve change within the group. (Healy 2005: 81)

Thus, Healy explains, reactive emotions that lead to viewing all care providers as acting self-interestedly fail not only to recognise the different attitudes and approaches amongst providers, but also the sometimes complex structures, directives and constraints within which they work (Healy 2005: 81; see also Healy 2000). As such, that which seems essential for promoting inclusion ends up with a divisive and reactive response.

Healy's account of *ressentiment* appears to conclude with the familiar social work themes of good communication and inclusive dialogue: avoid caricaturing the 'powerful', and they are more likely to listen to voices from the margins (2005: 82). Rights-based discourses are, after all, resolved through reaching a consensual agreement on how best to recognise and uphold the most relevant rights.[3] Nietzsche's point, however, is not to express a mere aversion to 'oppositional' politics. Rather, it is the values that reactive forces produce which come to dominate not just our morality, but our sense of both identity and interpretation as well. The danger, for both Nietzsche and his contemporary interpreters, is that an identity structured by *ressentiment* either misdirects or limits the extent to which one thinks outside of the governing systems of rights, justice or morals:

> Whereas all noble morality grows out of a triumphant saying 'yes' to itself, slave morality says 'no' on principle to everything that is 'outside', 'other', 'non-self': and this 'no' is its creative deed. This reversal of the evaluating glance – this *inevitable* orientation to the outside instead of back onto itself – is a feature of *ressentiment*. (Nietzsche 1997: 20)

This leads, Nietzsche argues, to interpretations of identity as something 'fixed' or 'essential'.[4] The capacity for a person to re-interpret the world around them is limited so long as they are working within reactive forces. Hence, the reactive identity focuses on their disempowerment, and looks for a system of morality which will bring down those more powerful who inflict suffering on them. In Brown's words, 'in its attempt to displace suffering, identity structured by *ressentiment* at the same time becomes invested in its own subjection' (1995: 70). The active identity, meanwhile, looks to the broader conditions of this relationship as contingent, historical and changeable; and in doing so, unearths the deeper roots of the power imbalance. This is the more difficult path, for Nietzsche, because it involves recognising that there are no immediate facts to appeal to, but only interpretations; and no 'moral phenomena, only a moral interpretation of the phenomena' (Nietzsche 2002: 64).

Thinking through Practice

Writing from a Marxist (rather than Nietzschean) perspective, Ferguson *et al.* have challenged the 'almost unchallengeable "common sense" within critical social policy and social work thought' that the dominant group benefit from the oppression of a minority (2002: 104). Instead, they argue that discrimination serves only to promote forms of what Nietzsche might term reactive morality. Stigmatising mental health problems, for example, makes people afraid to identify or seek help for their own mental health issues. In turn, there is a failure to address the root causes of such issues, which may well involve embedded socio-cultural expectations of 'normality' connected to oppressive systems of work or over-idealised norms of the family life.

Would you agree with Ferguson *et al.*'s argument here? To what extent do you think this resonates with Nietzsche's critique of *ressentiment*?

It is possible, of course, to simply reject Nietzsche's concept of *ressentiment* outright: to reject that policies of inclusion are driven by the clumsy language of 'revenge', to affirm the value of compassion as an immovable principle of social care, or to challenge the idea that identity politics cannot be forward-looking (for such a challenge, see Weir 2008). But the value of Nietzsche's polemic is not just a preliminary psychological account of the role of emotions in the formation of identity and values (as has been the focus of its influence in European social theory); it is rather, I think, a healthy scepticism surrounding the platitudes of inclusion, which presses us to think about the ways in which subjects and voices 'appear' within social work knowledge, which involves articulating the relationship between the identities social work engages in, and the interpretative practices that frame them. The concept of *ressentiment*, and its production from reactive and active perspectives, is both a way of illuminating the tensions of framing marginalised identity within social work, *and* a critique to be responded to.

A politics of reaction: framing the voice

Let's return to where we started out: how might Price and Simpson's critique of the *Valuing People* policy respond to Nietzsche's challenge?

Firstly, we might see the policy *itself* as enacting a particular reactive agenda. In part, this is linked to the 'triumvirate' of influences that led to its implementation.

The campaigning voices of people with disabilities have highlighted how the notion of 'care' is frequently a tool of disempowerment; yet in doing so, as Barnes (2006) notes, they have also often accepted a dichotomy between dependence and autonomy. Not only does this mean that social care professionals have often figured the successful outcome of an 'independent lifestyle' as the ability for the service user to do it alone (see Leece and Peace 2010), it also contributes to the 'rejection of care *per se* in favour of a rights-based approach to support for disabled people', which has 'sometimes been couched in terms which are dismissive both of care as a social good and of those who provide it – both paid and unpaid' (Barnes 2006: 146–7). This echoes what Wendy Brown describes as the *ressentiment* which the liberalism of Western modernity carries. Similar to Foucault (who also drew heavily on Nietzsche's genealogical method), Brown suggests it is the excessive focus on individualism within such liberalism – individualism which affirms our identity as marked out in terms of its difference from others – that provides a 'false autonomy' for marginalised identities, which is 'also their vulnerability' (1995: 19). The move to re-cast service users as 'consumers' involves re-structuring their identity not just in terms of their access to service provision, but also in terms of a set of ideals and values regarding freedom, choice and power. Furthermore, the move to improve social care practices becomes embroiled within an assault on the premise of social care itself.

As Barnes argues, 'because independence is valued and care-giving is not, the interdependence which characterises all human life and which for everyone at some stage of their life is expressed through care, is not recognised' (Barnes 2006: 147); which Price and Simpson similarly found with the devaluing of carer roles in the implementation of *Valuing People*. They point to the fact that in two of their case studies, the 'independence' of Direct Payments is 'tempered by a continued "dependence" upon family, and a shifting of risk from state to family' (2009: 183), which is crucially obscured in the drive towards liberal autonomy. In this way, Brown argues that the subject of liberal reforms (such as *Valuing People*) remains paradoxical: 'it is their situatedness within power, and their production by power, and liberal discourse's denial of this situatedness and production that cast the liberal subject into failure' (1995: 67).

Thinking through Practice

In their article on perceptions of social policy amongst UK voters, Hoggett *et al.* (2013) argue that policy agendas based on the ideal of 'fairness' can in fact engender rivalries and competition between disadvantaged groups. In their research in white working class communities, they found that a sense of loss (of identity, community, or rights) was accompanied by a bitterness towards those 'others' who were perceived to benefit from welfare services. Rather than focus on the assault on welfare budgets that has followed the global financial crisis of 2008, the consequent lack of funding for projects such as social housing, or the problem of the 'living wage' (whereby those in work are still required to draw benefits) in general, Hoggett *et al.* found that their research

> participants instead wanted more conditions on benefits being received, based on a 'restricted and localized vision of injustice', echoing the nineteenth-century mantra of the 'deserving' and 'undeserving' poor. The authors thus argue:
>
>> Such a reactionary politics of grievance feeds off and amplifies *ressentiment*, an underlying structure of feeling, a matrix of toxic sentiments which, as our research indicates, sinks deep into the pores of civil society. These anti-social sentiments fracture solidaristic ties between people placed in the same powerless structural position in society. (Hoggett et al. 2013: 6)
>
> What do you think is the role – if any – of social work in addressing such an 'underlying structure of feeling'?

In many ways this reminds me of Stefan Dolgert's argument (2010) as to why structural analyses of marginalisation are so difficult to motivate active resistance to, because they are not 'seen' in the same way that liberal resentment can be: structures of oppression are ontologically real but politically false; enemies are ontologically false but politically real.

It is not surprising, then, that for Nietzsche reactive power produces a set of values which serve to regulate and enforce the dominant attitudes and sentiments of a society, but which ultimately always *fail* to materialise. This is part of the deep-rooted reactivity which structures liberal morality. Traditional moral theories such as utilitarianism (with its concern for the 'greater good') or Kantian deontology (with its concern for universal imperatives) are premised on projections of how the world *should* be. This is the key to their appeal, Nietzsche suggests, because they allow their proponents to 'cope' with the existing inequalities they suffer. But no such world is ever forthcoming, because they are based on fundamentally misleading premises: they suggest that the messy, intricate and unbalanced world of the present can be superseded by a 'true' world that lies in the future. For Nietzsche, such a desire for a singular truth is itself a part of the 'slave morality': it stems from an inability to confront the reality of inequalities and perspectival existence. 'The truthful man […] *thus affirms another* world from the one of life, nature and history' (2002: 112), and this 'will to truth' is nothing less than an expression of reactive power.

There are two implications for Nietzsche's critique, here. The first is that morality as a whole is doomed: a path which social workers are unlikely to find appealing, even if some may appreciate the 'important corrective to […] liberal optimism' (MacIntyre 1998: 215). We can perhaps leave this to one side. The second is that the search for a singular or true 'meaning' to injustice or inequality – *whose* fault is it? *who* is to blame? – can end up overlooking the more complex realities of marginalised horizons. Reactive identity is borne from reactive interpretation that refuses to recognise the contingency and historicity of those terms that the personalisation agenda employs so frequently – such as family, home, community and so on – in favour of projected ideals. Hence, Price and Simpson's case studies of service users within the *Valuing People* policy not only report how residential provisions for individuals with learning disabilities are closed at a greater speed than adequate alternate supports for medium to long-term care are appearing (2009: 185), but also 'show how the drive towards supported or community based provision can result in greater levels of vulnerability', and 'reveal that the "utopia" upon which the policy draws is far removed from the harshness of much of contemporary society': for example, once within the 'community', one service user experiences sexual exploitation; another financial exploitation at the hands of a loan shark (2009: 184). This interpretative aspect is important for laying the ground for an awareness of, and advocating for, service user voices that are 'active', and not 'reactive', or structured by *ressentiment*.

Interpreting identity: the challenge of listening

We may recall the argument earlier from both Fook and McLaughlin that the identity of the 'service user' was created through a relationship between a person and the services they engaged with. But while this relationship may raise a potential problem for essentialising the service user, and defining them in terms of their deficiencies or needs, it is also the basis of a dialogical relationship through which the problem of marginalised identity presents itself. It is, in other words, the basis of the fusion of horizons through which, according to Gadamer at least, understanding can take place as a transformative, rather than confirmative, venture.

This is the second point that I think Price and Simpson's work on *Valuing People* raises in response to Nietzsche. Each of their case studies highlights the contingency and historicity of the way in which service users come to be identified as such. The narratives show how marginalised identity is formed through unfolding paths, based on their relations with different personal and structural forms of 'care'. In this way, the distinctive situations of each service user provide a rich context for understanding how their 'voice' is articulated and produced, not simply as a voice itself, but the larger structure regarding the way in which it is heard or not heard. Indeed, Gayatri Spivak has argued, in the context of identifying marginal or 'subaltern' identities within postcolonial critiques (see Chapter 7), 'the question "Who should speak?" is less crucial than "Who will listen?"' (Spivak 1990: 59). This is, I think, something which seems more like an 'active' approach to identity that provides an alternative to Nietzsche's pessimism.

Writing in a different context, Kelly Oliver has argued that Nietzsche's concept of active and reactive force can also be applied to interpretation. Reactive interpretation, she argues, 'assumes that words are transparent windows onto [...] meaning'. Reactive forces, we will recall, see meaning as simply 'there', in a direct correlation of cause and effect; it is this which leads to a perpetual sense of powerlessness, as the 'causes' are typically abstract or beyond the reach of those who are affected. Active interpretation, meanwhile, 'involves a recognition of the investment the reader makes in the text's meaning and diagnoses the symptoms of that investment' (Oliver 1995: 19–20). While Oliver refers here to textual interpretation, the same notion can be applied to the dialogical situation involving the marginalised voice. This means that, while there is a clear importance for 'empirical research' to inform discussion surrounding policies aimed at increasing inclusion – research which is not as abundant as it might be (see Sims and Cabrita Gulyurtlu 2014) – a corresponding importance is attached to the interpretative frameworks being applied. Simply presenting empirical evidence of what service users have said or done will always risk being read representatively; which is why Roger Smith notes that 'it is the reification of terms, and the "taken-for-granted" nature of the language used' within practice 'which must be a central focus of the social work task' (2008: 164). If marginalised voices are to contest the meaning of their marginalisation – challenging the justice of their disempowerment, and questioning the context of their disadvantage – then the fullest structure of what 'meaning' means must be considered.

Numerous researchers attempting to find voices for the traditionally 'voiceless' have often found that marginalisation can run far deeper than the simple topography of moving those on the 'outside' to the 'inside'. To take some examples from outside of the personalisation context discussed thus far: Caroline Leeson's work on young people's access to decision-making highlights the expectation some adults have in seeking to protect children in care. Such children can be viewed as particularly vulnerable, which 'can create a situation where their voice is not heard and possibly render them more vulnerable, as they are not represented.' The desire to 'protect children from distress' frequently obscures the possible implications that 'the child feels further unable to express their wishes and feelings in relation to past events' (2007: 274). However, as Leeson goes on to note, this is not simply a case of assuming children possess the same power of articulation as adults. Rather, 'the onus is on adults to ensure children feel comfortable and familiar with the decision-making process engaged in to aid their participation, rather than make assumptions about age and competence' (275). Understanding needs instead to be 'co-constructed' (269), for which Leeson's own research uses 'layers of method' (275) rather than relying on one form of interview or exercise. In a different client context, Val Clark's discussion on the mutual aid practices she used in her work with asylum seekers in Australia (2006) shows how an 'open forum' model of group work can be used to challenge both the top-down approach to service provision (whereby the social worker holds knowledge, which the service user does not), and the traditional paternalistic focus on the individual 'case' of a service user. In this case, it is the concrete context in which the voice of the service user is heard (i.e. the interaction between facilitation, attendance and purposiveness of the forum) which transfigures both the social worker's own horizon (by, for example, adjusting their expectations of what they can 'hear' in a discussion, owing to the language capabilities of the participants), while also allowing the asylum seekers to 'make sense' of the challenges they faced, showing 'the capacity of [such] groups to unleash powerfully therapeutic forces of mutual aid and self-empowerment' (Clark 2006: 387). Clark's story is one of opening oneself up to the vulnerability of listening: as she reflects, it involved 'learning on the run, trial and error and constant refinement of my thinking' in order for facilitation to be successful (383).

What strikes me about these two somewhat arbitrary examples of 'marginalised voices' is the way in which the emergence of the marginalised voice almost always carries with it a *critique* of the ways in which we go about listening. This is not simply a case of a narrow dichotomy between the 'good' social worker who listens out for different perspectives, and the 'bad' social worker who relentlessly and unreflectively pursues the habits they always have. As Fook notes, the act of listening is often framed by discursive and interpretative assumptions which, once embedded, are difficult to shift. In contrast, these examples question the presumption that a single 'truth' dominates the scene of marginalisation, which is substituted with another if the service user's voice is heard. Instead, they widen the possible meanings ascribed to a policy or process. This is not opening up the scene to a limitless relativism, however, whereby all perspectives are equal, and nor is it determining that each individual – social worker, care provider, asylum seeker, young person in care etc. – speaks from some fixed, core perspective. Rather, in recognising the contingency of an identity, the *conditions* of that contingency – the historical, moral, political and social reasons for this interpretative relationship (or fusion of horizons) coming into place – are brought to the fore. This is perhaps why, in Crossley and Crossley's words, the history of any social rights movement 'is always, in part, a history of the reconfiguration of habitus' (2001: 1487). And perhaps this is the resonance of our short word from Nietzsche: that a politics of marginalised identity must be one of *transfiguration*, and not domination (see Strong 1975); active, and not reactive.

But both Clark and Leeson's research – which shares no other similarities other than a focus on otherwise silenced or concealed perspectives – can be read as performing what Fook calls an 'act of *reconstruction*' in order for 'marginalised and silenced perspectives to be heard'; which involves 'negotiating the ways in which discourses are heard and expressed' (Fook 2002: 97). In what Fook terms 'contextual practice', she argues that social workers need the 'ability to recognise simultaneous multiple positions and perspectives […] [which] allows the ability to work *with* whole contexts, while at the same time working within them' (2002: 144, emphasis original). Unlike reactive interpretation, that fixates upon single 'truths' of situations, whereby marginalisation is reduced to being the *fault* of an individual, or caused by the state, and so on, Fook asserts that within an active contextual practice 'the emphasis is on *elucidating meaning* rather than *preserving the "truth"*' (146).

Price and Simpson's critique of *Valuing People* raises the problem of how progressive agendas for change can come to be dominated by specific political or economic interests. In response, what their case studies offer is less a series of voices that 'speak for themselves' – each case is certainly lamentable, but not voyeuristically so – and more a complex contestation of the ways in which key terms in the agenda are *interpreted*: such as, autonomy, rights, individuality and self-development. When they conclude that it is 'an indictment of current policy implementation that little has been learned from previous experience', and that this has led to a familiar 'set of "unintended consequences" from progressive policy aims' (2009: 185), it highlights the need not just for better representation of marginalised identities, but better listening and interpretation on the part of those within the 'centre'.

Thinking through Practice

It is worth noting that Fook's account of contextual practice has been criticised by many for its 'postmodern' approach, which removes a clear sense of politics, and leads to relativism and conceptual inconsistencies (Pease 2013: 25).

Could a case be made, then, that radical or critical forms of social work in fact *require* some kind of *ressentiment* in order to be effective in their structural critiques of oppression? Is there more to be said for reactive force than Nietzsche gives credit to?

Notes

1 Nietzsche is in many senses a philosopher like no other, and while there is not the space here for a full treatment of his style of philosophy, some words of caution may be necessary. As I have argued elsewhere:

> Nietzsche's style of arguing is at once rigorously philological, tracing the historical development of concepts with intense academic skill, and at the same time almost hopelessly generalizing, aiming broad shots across the bows of our expectations of what a philosophical argument should be. This style must be borne in mind when approaching the logic of Nietzsche's argument [...] [It] is far more a polemic than it is an exercise in close reasoning, and at least one of its aims is to open our eyes to a world without fixed parameters of meaning and truth, and in its place, a raw flux of energy and power. (Grimwood 2011: 53)

2 Peter Sloterdijk (2000, cited in Halsall 2005) has used the terms 'horizontal communication' and 'vertical communication' to similar effect, though with less provocative language, in order to differentiate communication that draws distinctions between cultural values – the lived experience of the service user as a political critique, rather than the reflection of a determined, fixed identity ('but *of course* they were always going to say that...'), and the idea that no such distinctions are possible, as no one perspective can be said to be superior to others.

3 This implicit model of consensus has been criticised by Rancière for failing to account for the interplay of privilege at work in them. He argues that consensus is the 'reduction of democracy to the way of life of a society', and because this shrinks the space for any political discussion, political rights themselves begin to 'appear actually empty'. It is on this condition, he cynically suggests, that minority rights begin to be recognised: for once rights 'seem to be of no use [...] you do the same as charitable persons do with their old clothes. You give them to the poor' (Rancière 2004: 306–7).

4 The cultural theorist Michel de Certeau echoes Nietzsche with his argument regarding the emergence of group identities based on 'cultural' differences:

> A cultural, social, or ethnic autonomy always draws attention to itself by saying no: No, says the black, I am not American. No, says the Indian, I am not a Chilean or an Argentinian. [...] That is an absolutely basic beginning, but it very quickly becomes deceptive if we stick to it, since we risk identifying both with a political ideology and an exclusively cultural formation (de Certeau 1997: 69).

De Certeau argues that, because minorities have no political power (hence why they are minorities), they are effectively limited to ideology and discourse, the manner of which is already shaped by dominant forces. This is a problem, de Certeau thinks, because the cultural expressions they rely on are 'only the surface of a social unity that has not yet been given its own political and cultural consistency' (1997: 69).

References

Barnes, M. (2006). *Caring and Social Justice*. Basingstoke: Palgrave Macmillan.
Behuniak, S. (2011). 'The Living Dead? The Construction of People with Alzheimer's Disease as Zombies.' *Aging & Society*, 31, 70–92.
Beresford, P. (2005). 'Social Approaches to Madness and Distress: User Perspectives and User Knowledges.' In Tew, J. (ed.), *Social Perspectives in Mental Health*. London: Jessica Kingsley Publishers, pp. 32–52.
Brown, W. (1995). *States of Injury: Power and Freedom in Late Modernity*. Princeton, NJ: Princeton University Press.
—— (2006). *Regulating Aversion: Toleration in the Age of Empire*. Princeton, NJ: Princeton University Press.
Burton M. and Kagan C. (2006). 'Decoding Valuing People.' *Disability and Society*, 21, 4, 299–313.
Clark, V. (2006). 'Group Work Practice with Australia's Asylum Seekers.' *Australian Social Work*, 59, 4, 378–90.
Clarke, J. (2004). *Changing Welfare, Changing States: New Directions in Social Policy*. London: Sage.
Connolly, W. (1988). *Political Theory and Modernity*. Oxford: Basil Blackwell.
Connolly, W. (2002). *Identity/Difference: Democratic Negotiations of Political Paradox*. Minneapolis: University of Minnesota Press.
Cree, V. and Davis, A. (2006). *Social Work: Voices from the Inside*. London: Routledge.
Crossley, M. and Crossley, N. (2001). 'Patient Voices, Social Movements and the Habitus: How Psychiatric Survivors Speak Out.' *Social Science & Medicine*, 52, 10, 1477–89.
Dalrymple, J. and Burke, B. (1995). *Anti-Oppressive Practice: Social Care and the Law*. Maidenhead: Open University Press.
De Certeau, M. (1997). *Culture in the Plural*, T. Conley (trans.). Minneapolis, MN: University of Minnesota Press.
Deleuze, G. (2006 [1962]). *Nietzsche and Philosophy*, Tomlinson, H. (trans.). London: Continuum.
Dolgert, S. (2010). 'In Praise of Ressentiment: Or, How I Learned to Stop Worrying and Love Glenn Beck.' *APSA 2010 Annual Meeting Paper*. Available at SSRN: http://ssrn.com/abstract=1642232
Dominelli, L. (2004). *Social Work: Theory and Practice for a Changing Profession*. Cambridge: Polity Press.
Ferguson, I. (2008). *Reclaiming Social Work: Challenging Neo-Liberalism and Promoting Social Change*. London: Sage.
Ferguson, I., Lavalette, M. and Mooney, G. (2002). *Rethinking Welfare: A Critical Perspective*. London: Sage.
Fook, J. (2002). *Social Work: Critical Theory and Practice*. London: Sage.
Gadamer, H-G. (1999). *Hermeneutics, Religion and Ethics*, J. Weinsheimer (trans.). London: Yale University Press.
—— (2004). *Truth and Method*, J. Weinsheimer (trans.). London: Continuum.
Grimwood, T. (2011). 'Nietzsche and the Death of God.' In Bruce, M. and Barbone, S. (eds.), *Just the Arguments: 100 of the Most Important Arguments in Western Philosophy*. Oxford: Wiley Blackwell, pp. 52–6.
Halsall, R. (2005). 'Sloterdijk's theory of Cynicism, Ressentiment and "Horizontal Communication".' *International Journal of Media and Cultural Politics*, 1, 2, 163–79.
Hanley, B., Bradburn, J., Barnes, M., Evans, C., Goodare, H., Kelson, M., Kent, A., Olivers, A., Thomas, S. and Wallcraft, J. (2004). *Involving the Public in NHS Public Health and Social Care: Briefing Notes for Researchers*. Eastleigh: Involve.

Hans, J. (1992). *Contextual Authority and Aesthetic Truth*. Albany, NY: State University of New York Press.

Harding, S. (1991). *Whose Science? Whose Knowledge? Thinking from Women's Lives*. New York: Cornell University Press.

Healy, K. (1999). 'Power and Activist Social Work.' In Pease, B. and Fook, J. (eds.), *Transforming Social Work Practice*. London: Routledge, pp.115–34.

—— (2000). *Social Work Practices: Contemporary Perspectives on Change*. London: Sage.

—— (2005). *Social Work Theories in Context: Creating Frameworks for Practice*. Basingstoke: Palgrave.

Hoggett, P., Wilkinson, H. and Beedell, P. (2013). 'Fairness and the Politics of Resentment.' *Journal of Social Policy*, 42, 1, 1–9.

Jones, C. (2004). 'The Neo-Liberal Assault: Voices from the Front-line of British State Social Work.' In Ferguson, I., Lavalette, M. and Whitmore, E. (eds.), *Globalisation, Global Justice and Social Work*. London: Routledge, pp. 97–108.

Le Doeuff, M. (1989). *The Philosophical Imaginary*. C. Gordon (trans.). London: The Athlone Press.

Leece J. and Peace S. (2010). 'Developing New Understandings of Independence and Autonomy in the Personalised Relationship.' *British Journal of Social Work*, 40, 1847–65.

Leeson, C. (2007). 'My Life in Care: Experiences of Non-participation in Decision-Making Processes.' *Child and Family Social Work*, 12, 268–77.

MacIntyre, A. (1998 [1967]). *A Short History of Ethics*. London: Routledge.

McLaughlin, H. (2007). 'What's in a Name?: "Client", "Patient", "Customer", "Consumer", "Expert by Experience", "Service User" – What's Next?', *British Journal of Social Work*, 39, 6, 1101–17.

—— (2012). *Understanding Social Work Research*. 2nd edn. London: Sage.

Meltzer, B. and Musolf, G. (2002). 'Resentment and Ressentiment.' *Sociological Inquiry*, 72, 2, 240–55.

Mitchell, G., Dupuis, S. and Kontos, P. (2013). 'Dementia Discourse: From Imposed Suffering to Knowing Other-Wise.' *Journal of Applied Hermeneutics*, 1–19.

Morris, J. (2001). 'Impairment and Disability: Constructing an Ethics of Care that Promotes Human Rights.' *Hypatia*, 16, 4, 1–16.

Nietzsche, F. (1997 [1887]). *On the Genealogy of Morality*. C. Diethe (trans.). Cambridge: Cambridge University Press.

—— (2002 [1886]). *Beyond Good and Evil*. J. Norman (trans.). Cambridge: Cambridge University Press.

Oliver, K. (1995). *Womanizing Nietzsche: Philosophy's Relation to the 'Feminine'*. London: Routledge.

Parker, S., Fook, J. and Pease, B. (1999). 'Empowerment: The Modernist Social Work Concept Par Excellence.' In Pease, B. and Fook, J. (eds.), *Transforming Social Work Practice*. London: Routledge, pp. 150–57.

Pease, B. (2013). 'A History of Critical and Radical Social Work.' In Gray, M. and Webb, S. (eds.), *The New Politics of Social Work*. Basingstoke: Palgrave Macmillan, pp. 21–43.

Potts, K. and Brown, L. (2008) 'Becoming an Anti-Oppressive Researcher.' In Webber, M. and Bezanson, K. (eds.), *Rethinking Society in the 21st Century: Critical Readings in Sociology*. Toronto: Canadian Scholars' Press, pp. 50–7.

Price, V. and Simpson, G. (2009). 'From Inclusion to Exclusion: Some Unintended Consequences of *Valuing People*.' *British Journal of Learning Disabilities*, 38, 180–6.

Rancière, J. (2004). 'Who is the Subject of the Rights of Man?' *The South Atlantic Quarterly*, 103, 2, 297–310.

—— (2011). *The Politics of Aesthetics*. G. Rockhill (trans.). London: Continuum.
Rawls, J. (1971). *A Theory of Justice*. Cambridge, MA: Harvard University Press.
Sapiro, V. (1998). 'When are Interests Interesting?' In Phillips, A. (ed.), *Feminism and Politics*. Oxford: Clarendon Press, pp. 161–93.
Scheler, M. (1992). *On Feeling, Knowing, and Valuing: Selected Writings*. Chicago, IL: University of Chicago Press.
Schrift, A. (1990). *Nietzsche and the Question of Interpretation*. London: Routledge.
Scott, J. (1997). 'Deconstructing Equality-Versus-Difference: Or, the Uses of Poststructuralist Theory for Feminism.' In Tietjens Meyers, D. (ed.), *Feminist Social Thought: A Reader*. London: Routledge, pp. 757–70.
Sims, D. and Cabrita Gulyurtlu, S. (2014). 'A Scoping Review of Personalisation in the UK: Approaches to Social Work and People with Learning Disabilities.' *Health and Social Care in the Community*, 22, 1, 13–21.
Smith, A. (1977 [1776]). *An Inquiry into the Nature and Causes of the Wealth of Nations*. Chicago, IL: University of Chicago Press.
Smith, R. (2008). *Social Work and Power*. Basingstoke: Palgrave Macmillan.
Spivak, G.C. (1990). *The Post-Colonial Critic: Interviews, Strategies, Dialogues*. London: Routledge.
Strong, T. (1975). *Friedrich Nietzsche and the Politics of Transfiguration*. Los Angeles, CA: University of California Press.
Taylor, C. (1995). *Philosophical Arguments*. Harvard, MA: Harvard University Press.
Thornton, M. (2000). 'Neo-Liberalism, Discrimination and the Politics of Ressentiment.' In Jones, M. and Basser Marks, L. (eds.), *Explorations on Law and Disability in Australia*. Sydney: The Federal Press, pp. 8–27.
Weir, A. (2008). 'Global Feminism and Transformative Identity Politics.' *Hypatia*, 23, 4, 110–33.
Wilson, A. and Beresford, P. (2000). '"Anti-oppressive Practice": Emancipation or Appropriation?' *British Journal of Social Work*, 30, 5, 553–73.
Žižek, S. (2011). 'Afterword.' In Rancière, J. (ed.), *The Politics of Aesthetics*. G. Rockhill (trans.). London: Continuum, pp. 69–79.

4
ETHICS
Three concerns about human rights

Human rights in question

When the Universal Declaration of Human Rights (UDHR) was first published in 1948, it spoke as both a response to the moral demands of the humanitarian catastrophes of the Second World War, and a promise of the new world that emerged from the ruins. As the Preamble outlines, 'whereas disregard and contempt for human rights have resulted in barbarous acts which have outraged the conscience of mankind', the new Declaration brought forward 'a world in which human beings shall enjoy freedom of speech and belief and freedom from fear and want'. The Declaration was the product of international discussions, with the International Association of Schools of Social Work (IASSW) contributing to discussions throughout (Dominelli 2010: 99). It is not surprising, then, that it addresses some of the key tensions that social work encounters, particularly between the provision of service and the availability of resource, and between individual agency and the wider apparatus of the state. The Declaration itself sought to lay a foundation for the protection of individuals against abuse of political, legal or social power by establishing principles that went beyond specific political, legal or social systems. An individual's human rights enable them to challenge or resist the state they may otherwise be dependent upon. Hence, the content of the UDHR focuses on the freedom, protection, dignity and benefit of those who hold them (Beitz 2009).

Small wonder, then, that Social Work values are routinely linked to the principles of human rights. Most notably, the IASSW and International Federation of Social Work (IFSW) shared Statement of Ethical Principles declares that 'Principles of human rights and social justice are fundamental to social work'.[1] Much of contemporary social work practice is grounded on – implicitly or explicitly – a model of human rights. The nature of this grounding is not always agreed upon: whether, for example, human rights are employed as a *conceptual* framework for underpinning social work practice (Witkin 1998); or because rights-based practice is recognised as good professional *practice* (Reichert 2011); or because practitioners can utilise human rights as an international *instrument* to enhance the rights of citizens (Dominelli 2010); or even because human rights occupy a privileged position within the *discourse* of rights in general, grounded in the relationship between the discursive construction of rights and the applied practice of rights (Ife 1997, 2012). Human rights are fundamental; but in what sense they are fundamental is the question I want to address here.

> **Thinking through Practice**
>
> The 1948 UDHR begins by proclaiming that human rights are *endowed* to us. Do you think that human rights are something integral to individuals (i.e. something that we just 'have'), or something that is *given* or provided by a state, a law – or even a social worker?

At their most basic, human rights are things that everyone, everywhere, at every time, possess. They are *inalienable*: which does not mean they cannot, in practice, be overridden, but rather that one does not lose them or give them away. Thus, if these rights are denied to an individual, then there exists a moral imperative to enable that individual to reassert their rights. Furthermore, while some have argued that all of these rights should be reducible to one clear principle, such as individual freedom or dignity, with the individual articles being specific developments of a general theme (see Dworkin 2011), the human rights listed in the UDHR nevertheless cover a range of activities and interests, from interpersonal relationships to access to social services; from the right to participate in politics to the right to leisure time. Hence, human rights discourse can be apparent at the level of individual interaction (see, for example, Evans *et al.* (2012) on the application of human rights to service delivery for people with intellectual disabilities), or at the broader level of policy; for example, poverty eradication (George 2003) or environmental protection (Dominelli 2012). But more than this, as Witkin (1998) argues, human rights are in fact a multivalent tool for social work practice. The uses of human rights include giving social workers legitimacy to challenge the state and its treatment of disadvantaged individuals; promoting a universalist view of social justice, balanced with a relativist focus on human needs. Human rights maintain the importance of difference in persons and context, and their application supersedes any conflict between needs and merits. McDonald argues that they are 'an *unambiguous* and *inspiring morality* and politics for practitioners made despondent by the harshness and intractability of the contemporary workfare state' (McDonald 2006, my emphasis). It is this unambiguous legitimacy which underlies the egalitarian nature of Human Rights, and this can be used in turn to identify and challenge any disempowering processes within social work practice.

At the same time, it is precisely this notion of Human Rights as 'unambiguous and inspiring' that has caused some to raise questions over their use and understanding. The moment that an ethical basis or legal framework ceases to be questionable – either by virtue of becoming 'just common sense', or by standing atop unassailable moral heights – is the same moment that we lose the ability to critically discern appropriate use from inappropriate. As such, there are three specific concerns regarding the philosophical underpinning of human rights, and their relationship to social work, which I want to explore in this chapter.

1. Are human rights actually universal? And in what sense? Far from representing a neutral set of fundamental values which should be available to all, critics have disputed the 'universal' basis of such values; the power relations that they promote and enforce; and their usefulness as an effective set of ethical norms. It is often charged, for example, that the rights proffered are not so much universal as 'European'. The UDHR was not created as a document which describes how things are, but was intended to enact change in the world; and any change carries with it a standpoint that propels such a change. While paying passing regard to these criticisms – Dominelli, for example, writes that 'despite criticisms of individualistic and Western conceptualisation', the UDHR was nevertheless 'ratified by all members of the UN' (2010: 99) – many social work theorists remain intent that human rights should remain unquestionably the absolute basis of social work and social care values. Sometimes this leads to a conflation of different sources of 'universality'. For example, are human rights guaranteed by the rulings of national and international law (such as the International Bill of Human Rights in 1976)? If so, then their existence depends upon particular legal and political institutions. But this would make them changeable, whereas their invocation within social work practice seems to be something stronger – an inspiring morality, for example. In turn, while human rights may seem to offer a base set of shared values regarding morality, there remains disagreement on both the content of what should be included within the Declaration itself, and on the principles which underlie it. Asking how universal is the Universal Declaration requires *situating* the moral demands of human rights, and the rationality behind such a demand.

2. How does the concept of human rights emerge, historically? The fact that the UDHR emerged after the Second World War can suggest it speaks from a distinctly modern agenda. The ethical model of human rights allows for both individual interest (and thus a pluralism that reflects contemporary society) and a base level of universal agreement on our fundamental requirements. However, the idea that human rights are things which simply 'exist', innately within each human being, can lead to a certain ahistorical conception of what these rights are, where they come from, and who or what authorises them. Critics of the current formulation (and application) of human rights have probed the idea that these simply 'exist' without any historical background. Even if the Declaration was drawn up from long consultation and deliberation, its expression follows a

framework and language used by both the American Declaration of Independence (1776) and the *Declaration des droits de l'homme* (1789). Reading the development of human rights within the much broader context of the history of rights is not something that social work literature tends to do (given that, initially at least, discussions of duty in Ancient Rome take us about as far away from the domain of practice as we could get). However, by examining the history of the concept, we can also consider the effect of that history on the formation of the concept. In turn, this enables us to further clarify the objections mentioned in the first concern above.

3. Moving from the historical to the present day, what value do human rights bring to the ethical framework of social work practice? We have noted how social workers were key participants in discussions over the content of the UDHR. But are rights as a form of morality the most appropriate for the issues and dilemmas social workers face in contemporary practice? In other words, even if the first two points can be answered affirmatively, there remains the question of whether individual rights should form the moral basis of social work activity (as opposed to, say, the legal basis alone). This point has been raised recently by Stephen Webb, in an article critiquing human rights as the vestiges of post-modern ideas regarding identity politics. But how fair is this critique? And if not human rights, then what?

If not human rights, then what…? And there's the rub. We should not fail to notice that critiquing human rights is a risky business, because it opens up a range of possible accusations before any argument has even been formed. If human rights are challenged, does this mean that we are condoning acts of atrocity? That we are advocating moral or cultural relativism? Or removing any authority from social work values? While these objections are all answered straightforwardly – the challenging of rights does not entail their complete destruction; nor does it imply that a moral vacuum be left in the place of their ruins; nor does it necessarily condemn social work's authority, given that the nature of this authority is far more ambiguous and multivalent than the sheer clarity of human rights discourse – such objections nevertheless raise a distinct problem with how the discourse of rights appears to us in the twenty-first century. In short, part of the difficulty is that human rights have become so ingrained in practice (and social work culture), they are in certain contexts unquestionable. This is why to question them is so often construed as questioning everything, and can only leave us with nothing. And this is, of course, precisely why the critical social worker needs to be alert to their basis. It is also why critiques often adopt somewhat polemical or exaggerated positions, in order to avoid the problems they raise being easily absorbed back into the very discourse they want to challenge. Webb is one such polemical voice, when he expresses his concern over 'a rapidly expanding textbook genre within social work illustrative of a dumbing down process in scholarship in the name of marketing a fashionable human rights and diversity perspective' (Webb 2009: 308). The aim of critiquing human rights is not, though, simply to criticise for the sake of criticism; but rather, to encourage those who defend their value-base in terms of the depth of the concept, rather than a superficial appeal to rights in their most readymade form. To this end, we can look at each of the three concerns raised in order.

First concern: are human rights universal?

Even at their very inception, disputes arose as to how universal the Universal Declaration could be. In 1947, the Saudi Arabian delegation argued that the UN Commission on Human Rights had 'for the most part taken into consideration only the standards recognised by Western civilisation' (quoted in Pagden 2003: 171). A similar concern was raised by the American Anthropological Association, whose statement in 1947 asked: 'How can the proposed Declaration be applicable to all human beings, and not be a statement of rights conceived only in terms of the values prevalent in the countries of Western Europe and America?' (1947: 539). Since then, the concern regarding the assumed universality of human rights has been raised from many different perspectives: for example, theorists, jurists and politicians from across a number of non-European areas (see Twining 2006). Controversial as the Senior Minister of Singapore's claim in the 1990s that human rights neglected 'Asian' values of kinship and community was, his was not a lone voice expressing an incompatibility between traditions of value and rights-based ethics. Human Rights have also been critiqued by Islamic groups and traditions, and, at least until recently, the Catholic Church; not to mention European and North American academics. 'What all these criticisms have in common,' Anthony Pagden argues, 'is their clear recognition of – and objection to – the fact that "rights" are cultural artefacts masquerading as universal, immutable values' (Pagden 2003: 172).

The reasons for this are clear enough, as Pagden describes:

> [T]he very notion of a translocal, transcultural human right only makes sense within the context of a conception of 'humanity,' and since humanity is, empirically, and for whatever historical reason, social, then it can, in effect, only make sense in the context of a given understanding of what a society should be. (2003: 192)

This raises a problem for social work organisations attempting to reconcile their ethical frameworks with the need for cultural awareness and/or competence. For example, until it was revised in 2012, the British Association of Social Workers' (BASW) Code of Ethics held that social workers would 'recognise the diversity within and among cultures and will recognise the impact of their own ethnic and cultural identity', at the same time as having a 'duty' to respect human rights. But given that rights and culture are (at least according to the criticisms above) so interrelated, this could result in conflict if someone's 'cultural identity' did not incorporate the principles of human rights. In the revised (and much-improved) code, the language of duty was replaced by one of responsibility, and 'cultural identity' was replaced by the norm of offering services in a 'culturally appropriate manner'.

Before we examine this claim that human rights are cultural artefacts, however, we need to look at what we might term the liberal critique of rights. From this perspective, the claim that the full UDHR reflects universal principles is almost certainly flawed. This can, however, be redressed by adjusting the specific content of which Articles of the Declaration constitute human rights, and which are subsidiaries or added extras. For example, both Rawls (1971) and Cranston (1973) argue that particular Articles are more fundamental than others in the Declaration. For these thinkers, the core principles of human rights are fundamental to both human well-being, and universal justice. However, once we move beyond a certain point within the Declaration, the nature of the Articles moves beyond this into socially and culturally specific claims. So, for Rawls, Article 3 (the right to life, liberty and security) and Article 5 (the protection from harm) form the foundation of his political philosophy; whereas Article 22 (regarding the right to social security) begins to presume a certain kind of ordering of society – that is, one which has a social security system – which goes beyond the core individual need described in the first articles, and in doing so problematizes the later articles' claim to be universal. For this very reason, Rawls ignores all of the articles past Article 19.

This is sometimes described as the problem of 'human rights inflation': as more and more objects become seen as matters of human rights, the less and less powerful the status of such rights becomes. Such an argument tends to see the UDHR in terms of two 'generations' of rights-claims: the 'first generation' rights are those of security, property, participation and, above all, freedom; whereas the 'second generation' regard entitlement to subsistence, welfare, leisure and culture (Orend 2003: 110). For Rawls, only first-generation rights are sufficient principles for 'human' rights; the others are more like 'social' rights: still important, of course, but not as universal as *human* rights should be. For Cranston, only first-generation rights are deserving of the status of human rights, meaning that the second-generation rights-claims (and, more recently, the 'third generation' of issues that have been claimed as matters of human rights – for example, self-determination of minority groups or new nations) are better understood as being goals to aim for, rather than actual fundamental conditions of human existence. This objection was realised in full when human rights were translated into International Law, where the civil and political rights were separated from the social rights. Added to this, thinkers such as James Nickel (2007) have argued that on a practical basis it would be almost impossible for the later generation rights-claims to be supported universally in both material and financial terms, given the disparities in wealth between countries across the world.

Thinking through Practice

Is 'human rights inflation' a genuine problem for social work practitioners? In what kinds of situations might there be a prospect of a service user having *too many* human rights?

For thinkers such as Rawls and Cranston, the universal *moral* imperative of human rights can remain, but as moral imperatives they exclude the more concrete and socio-cultural and political demands of the later Articles. These arguments raise a number of issues, though, regarding how we can effectively 'pick and choose' which rights are more important than others. Interestingly, in contrast, even a cursory glance at the research will show immediately that the application of human rights within social work makes much more use of the later articles, positioning them as utterly important to interventions in complex situations (see Wronka 1998). After all, having one's freedom and security is of no use if one is simultaneously denied basic healthcare or education. The first generation rights will remain only abstract ideals without some kind of material and social support; and given that this conflict between liberal ideals and restrictions on resources is one of the key tensions within the social work role, it is not surprising that social work theory tends not to draw the 'generational' distinction that the likes of Rawls do. Even in their most core form, it cannot be disputed that the rise of human rights, and their expression in the UDHR, arose from specific problems and contexts that demanded a response. As such, to look for some kind of 'clean' dividing line between the core sense of what it is to be human, and the socio-cultural surroundings of the human is unlikely to be successful. We need only revisit the debate between liberals and communitarians in the previous chapters to see this.

'Human', or 'Western'?

Given that human rights may almost necessarily also be socio-cultural, the problem then emerges as to which socio-cultural system is being presupposed. The answer here is often given clearly: the values that human rights represent emanate from distinctively 'European', or 'Western', or 'Capitalist', or 'Liberal' ideals. As Žižek recounts:

> 'Man', the bearer of human rights, is generated by a set of political practices which materialise citizenship; 'human rights' are, as such, a false ideological universality, which masks and legitimises concrete politics of Western imperialism, military interventions and neo-colonialism. (Žižek 2005: 128–9)

In response to this concern that human rights reflect Western values – a claim that is brought to light more fully by the historical analysis in the next section – thinkers from outside of, or critical of, the 'Western tradition' have given consensus-based, radical and progressive alternatives, which we can mention here, far too briefly.

A growing field of study on cross-cultural ethics looks for consensus on the content of human rights, whilst remaining sensitive to the need for political legitimacy and cultural context (see, for example, An-Na'im 1995; An-Na'im and Deng 1990; Charles Taylor has made a somewhat similar argument, which is discussed in Chapter 7). Such studies, of course, must pay careful attention to the risk of failing to identify the concrete space in which such 'cross-cultural consensus' takes place; not to mention the risk of essentialising certain practices or values as 'cultural' rather than historical or political. Radical writers such as the Islamist thinker Mawdudi (1976) have argued that the concept of human rights is poorly served by Western philosophical paradigms, as it remains too heavily influenced by the alignment of modern rationality and economic capitalism (the rights of the 'individual' are, in their current formulation by the UDHR, only really the rights of the consumer). Thinkers such as the feminist theologian Riffat Hassan,[2] meanwhile, have attempted to synthesise principles of human rights with Islamic traditions, by arguing that Qur'anic values underlie what the UDHR is attempting to achieve. This has led to alternative versions of the UDHR being drawn up. For example, the drafting of the Universal Islamic Declaration of Human Rights (UIDHR) in 1981 by the Islamic Council of Europe, was an attempt to maintain the ethos of the 1948 declaration, whilst redressing the issues that Muslim delegations had raised at the time of its writing. In particular, it engaged with two problematic areas: first, the model of individual freedom that the Declaration begins from (which reflects a specific philosophical approach to the self not necessarily shared in non-European cultures), and second, the anthropocentrism of the Declaration – in other words, the shaping of rights around the needs of man, rather than of God. For the Islamic Council of Europe, respect for the rights of fellow human beings is not only through law enforcement but also guarded by moral consciousness.[3] If human rights are to be seen as a moral demand, then they require a stronger moral framework than simple 'freedom'. Hence, the Preamble states: 'By terms of our primeval covenant with God our duties and obligations have priority over our rights.' The result is that, while the UIDHR maintains much of the general content of the UDHR, it situates this in terms of divine revelation as a definitive guide for law (this is, indeed, a constitutional principle in most Muslim countries).

Such alternative and counter-declarations are far from unproblematic, however. As Heiner Bielefeldt points out, if the significance of human rights lies in their very universality, then aligning them to one or another culture is dangerous: 'to divide the idea of human rights into "Western," "Islamic," and other culturally defined conceptions […] would be the end of universal human rights. The language of human rights would thus simply be turned into a rhetorical weapon for intercultural competition' (2000: 92). Yet, in many senses, this is precisely what is already happening. In the mainstream media today, human rights are frequently raised through cultural flashpoints: whether Muslim girls should wear the veil in French schools; or what role Shari'a law should have in Muslim communities residing in non-Muslim countries. If human rights discourse carries with it a demand for a particular kind of politics, community and identity, it would not be surprising if this were to create a *de facto* conflict with those who contested these. It is unsurprising, then, that alternative formulations of human rights are often seen as ways of covering up human rights abuses that are currently happening. But as Slavoj Žižek has argued, appeals to human rights within capitalist societies – appeals which would, of course, include those made by the social work theorists that we began by listing – rest on contradictory assumptions.

One such assumption is that human rights oppose fundamentalism; which here refers not just to its religious incarnation, but any discourse which naturalises or essentialises what are, in fact, contingent traits. For example, in cases where a service user's mental health capacity is being assessed, human rights are appealed to in order to maintain a focus on the dignity and need of the individual, rather than generic diagnostic categories: 'By classifying a person's thoughts and belief systems as "delusional" or "paranoid", or even by reducing their experiences to "symptoms" such as "anxious" or "depressed", mental health professionals can undermine a person's freedom of thought' (Forrest 2014: 32). By delivering services according to the principles of upholding rights, though, such categories can be challenged, and 'the other less easily measured themes of recovery as a personally defined and experienced process or journey, such as hope, acceptance and identity, are likely to follow' (Forrest 2014: 31–2). However, the problem with opposing fundamentalism as a 'naturalising' tendency is that it overlooks the 'naturalising' element within human rights *itself*. This echoes, ironically, Cranston's critique of 'third generation' rights claims which produce a politics based on different identities, rather than shared core principles. Žižek refers to this as 'an unprecedented re-naturalization' whereby public discussions of rights are more often than not 'now translated into attitudes towards the regulation of "natural" or "personal" idiosyncrasies' (2005: 117). This is, of course, a similar claim to Nancy regarding the 'retreat of politics', and what Alain Badiou has argued regarding identity politics, which is discussed below.

Žižek argues that this is enforced by the assumption within human rights-claims that the 'two most basic rights are freedom of choice, and the right to dedicate one's life to the pursuit of pleasure (rather than to sacrifice it for some higher ideological cause)' (2005: 115). But the notion of a freedom of choice is already conditioned by our expectation of what 'free choice' would appear to be; as Žižek illustrates, using the case of the veil:

> The problem of pseudo-choice [...] demonstrates the limitations of the standard liberal attitude towards Muslim women who wear the veil: acceptable if it is their own free choice rather than imposed on them by husbands or family. However, the moment a woman dons the veil as the result of personal choice, its meaning changes completely: it is no longer a sign of belonging to the Muslim community, but an expression of idiosyncratic individuality. In other words, a choice is always a meta-choice, a choice of the modality of the choice itself: it is only the woman who does not choose to wear a veil that effectively chooses a choice. (Žižek 2005: 118)

There is another way of viewing these hidden conditions of human rights, though. Thinkers such as Jack Donnelly have argued that, in fact, a Western liberal paradigm is *essential* for any emergence of human rights at all (Donnelly 1982), because human rights are a Western formulation of the universal aspiration for human *dignity*. In other words, the problem of universality arises from confusing two distinct terms: dignity, which Donnelly argues that all cultures hold as essential, and rights, which are particularly pertinent to Western societies, but not necessarily others. Different versions of this argument suggest that cultural difference does not *in itself* remove the importance of Human Rights as a moral ideal. They still have universal application by virtue of being a more worthy framework than the alternatives. Likewise, if the principles of Human Rights are accepted as a core value base – as they are in the most prominent international social work organisations – then it can be argued that these can only be realised within a certain set of political, cultural and relational practices.

This does not sidestep the issues, so much as call into question the value of liberalism as a way of conceiving of basic human rights in the first place. This can possess some serious internal contradictions. For example, Žižek notes that the liberal approach is dominated by the notion of 'negative liberty' – that is, that one is free to do what one wants, so long as it does not interfere with anyone else. In this way, he argues, 'liberal attitudes towards the other are characterized both by respect for otherness, openness to it, and an obsessive fear of harassment'. But if by 'respecting otherness' we only mean either those who are exactly like us, or those who keep their distance, in such a way that they are no bother or challenge, then this does not really seem to be 'toleration'. Žižek remarks: 'the other is welcomed insofar as its presence is not intrusive, *insofar as it is not really the other*. Tolerance thus coincides with its opposite' (2005: 120, my emphasis).

Thinking through Practice

To what extent do you think that these arguments surrounding human rights as an ethical basis regarding imperialism, hegemony and difference would *also* apply to other ethical theories that social work draws upon, which depend on 'universal' rules (such as Utilitarianism or Deontology)?

While differing in background, this kind of approach seems to be what Erika Haug has in mind when she criticises the notion of 'international social work' for explicitly stepping away from the commitments to particular and situated views in the name of objectivity. Instead, she suggests, social work should embrace the commitments that it begins from:

> If defined by a commitment to human rights and social justice, international social work involves challenging oppression at the individual, community, regional, national and international levels, guided by a clear vision of a more equitable global society. Thus, rather than playing an apolitical role […], the focus of ISW activities could be on anti-oppression practice, de-colonization, political advocacy and solidarity work by connecting 'communities of resistance.' (Haug 2005: 133)

For social work, then, the philosophical problem is not as simple as a choice between a naïve belief in universal rights on the one hand, and cultural relativism on the other. The problem is rather how the 'universality' is experienced on the ground level of practice, and to what extent the politics of this universality shapes its application. On the one hand, if human rights are a legacy of European imperialism, and should be contested rather than accepted, then the importance of culture in shaping our values and approaches needs to overrule the reliance on the core principles of the UDHR as the basis of social work ethics. On the other hand, it is possible to view human rights as essentially Eurocentric, yet still hold on to these values as worth pushing. In other words, it might be the case that adopting the principles of human rights allows for the most cultural competence, as opposed to understanding culture in order to arrive at principles. But to know which path to follow, we need a closer understanding of why human rights may be seen as fundamentally European.

Second concern: are human rights historical?

Human rights can often be invoked within a context of immanent demand. In the traditional ethical dilemmas that we find in social work textbooks, the emphasis is on decision-making within an often pressurised situation. The solidity of rights is their strength; and as such, exploring their historical contingency can often be seen as in some way undermining, or simply unnecessary.

But as we have discussed, human rights did not simply appear from out of nowhere. Given their emergence and acceptance within Western societies, Bielefeldt argues that 'there are good reasons to assume that the genesis of the idea of human rights can, in one way or another, be linked to the religious, philosophical, and cultural sources of [that] tradition' (Bielefeldt 2000: 92). Some, like Hugman, may go as far as acknowledging that the foundations of modern human rights are rooted in the work of Thomas Hobbes and John Locke in the seventeeth century, as they 'shared the view that human beings are naturally free and equal in a moral and political sense, and must find ways to agree on how to live together in ordered societies' (2013: 160). But this glosses over a number of deeper points regarding the differences between modern rights and what went before, and in particular Dalacoura's (2003) argument that the concept of human rights somewhat problematically merges two often opposing strands in Western philosophical and political thought: Natural Law and the Enlightenment.

In its classical formulations in the early centuries of the Common Era, natural law was simply the natural aptitudes of human beings (as well as animals) – eating, sleeping, reproducing, and so on. With the establishment of the Roman Empire across most of Europe and North Africa, however, there was a corresponding rise of cross-cultural disputes, where the increase in trade and migration meant that different local customs often came into conflict. Partly due to this, the notion of a law that applied to all people, regardless of culture, began to take form; which was, in very blunt terms, that by being part of the Roman society, one was obliged to behave according to certain public duties. By the thirteenth century, this had become perhaps the most influential version of natural law, embedded within medieval scholastic philosophy. This version asserts that 'human law is in some sense derived from moral norms that are universally valid and discoverable by reasoning about human nature' (Greenawalt 1987: 161). In other words, it sees 'law' and 'morality' as interchangeable (this is, in part, due to the history of the use of the term 'morality' itself, which only takes on the form that we currently use in around the eighteenth century (see MacIntyre 1998)). It sees the human sense of what is 'right' and 'wrong' as reflecting the natural order of the world, and the laws that govern it; which, in turn, are laid down by divine law. As the great medieval theologian, St. Thomas Aquinas, wrote in the thirteenth century: 'Every human law has just so much of the nature of law as it is derived from the law of nature. But if, in any point, it deflects from the law of nature [i]t is no longer a law but a perversion of law' (1954: 129). In this way, the organisation of society, the hierarchical systems of governance, and the principles of justice, all reflected the way that the world 'is'. It also meant that such laws contained a link between individual, society and universe which invoked a responsibility as much as it did a 'right'.

Within the period of time known as the Enlightenment, however, the contexts which underlay natural law were challenged. Theologically, the Protestant reformation in Europe challenged the Catholic interpretation of divine law; this suggested that rather than be 'revealed' to us, morality must be interpreted. Scientifically, the figures of Copernicus, Galileo, and Newton, all challenged the specific ordering of the universe that informed Natural Law theories. Politically, thinkers such as Hobbes, Grotius, and Rousseau provided alternative rationalities for deciding upon questions of right and wrong, based on human agreement on our 'Natural Rights' rather than revealed truth. Overall, the idea that the world speaks one single, natural truth to us is contested; and the fact that such a 'single truth' can only be achieved through violent suppression of alternative voices (as was demonstrated, first by the protestant reformation, and then by the European conquest of the New World) becomes evident.

Human rights, it is often held, emerge from a kind of collision of these two perspectives. The aftermath of the Second World War provides both an opportunity and a need for a new moral foundation to be laid which recognises the fundamental equality and dignity of the human being, regardless of society, culture or religion. Such a foundation cannot be based simply on the tools of existing moral theories – for example, utilitarianism – as the rational deliberation they require is too easily manipulated to suit the ends of the powerful. Human rights thus retain the idea, from natural law, that there is some kind of intrinsic morality that is, in effect, 'natural' to us, above and beyond the control of the state or society which we live in. But this notion of a common humanity is sufficiently distinct, due to the grounds laid by the Enlightenment – more rational, more empirical, less 'religious' – to constitute a viable moral agreement where natural law failed.

> **Thinking through Practice**
>
> Given the history leading up to their formulation, would you say that human rights are the most appropriate basis for social work ethics in the twenty-first century? Are there *significant* ethical differences between social work today and social work in 1948, in relation to shifts in culture and society?

This leaves some ambiguity, however. The 1948 declaration begins by proclaiming, are human rights *endowed* to us; an expression that has perhaps perpetuated the tension that human rights are both something integral to individuals, and something that can be *given* by a law, a state or even a social worker (see Oliver's critique of 'empowerment' in this regard (1990))? *Where* do human rights exist? Are they within us? Are they social institutions formed by discursive interaction? Are they, as Foucault might argue, techniques for identity formation?

Natural law and natural rights

The answer, in part, lies in specifying the exact relationship between human rights and natural law; and there is, as one might imagine, a range of different arguments regarding this. The key to the ambiguity lies in the shift from natural *law* to natural *rights*. Whereas natural law is embedded within a cosmological holism, whereby the individual is only given meaning or existence as part of the wider structure of world, the shift to natural rights inverts this relationship. In successive images – Hobbes, Locke and Rousseau's 'state of nature', Daniel Defoe's *Robinson Crusoe*, and so on – the world, and society within it, are seen as something effectively created by man's will. The rise of the individual is fundamental to the rise of rights; but this creates a problem for the very idea of a 'common humanity' that rights invoke for their authority.

For pre-modern thinkers such as Aquinas or Aristotle, self-preservation required sociability. People always lived within communities, and necessarily – they depended on them for the virtues of health, food, friendship, and protection. Self-preservation, as a natural instinct, was thus bound to a range of communal activities. For the early modern thinkers, such as Grotius and Hobbes, self-preservation is far simpler: self-preservation is not dying. Hence, Hobbes describes natural rights as briefly as:

> That which is not against our reason, men call RIGHT, or *jus*, or blameless liberty of using our own natural power and ability. It is therefore a *right of nature*: that every man may preserve his own life and limbs, with all the power he hath. (Hobbes 2008: 71)

The 'natural power and ability' is not tied to political membership of a localised community (*ius*), but rather as a rights-bearing individual. In this way, natural rights become increasingly subjective throughout the modern era; they are held by the subject, *as* a subject, and rights are relative to the rights-bearer, rather than external systems such as community, society or the world.

In this way, the notion of 'right' gradually loses its sense of obligation and responsibility, and is replaced with three conditions on which it draws authority. These are, in short, *property*, *contract* and *freedom*. The power of natural rights is, first and foremost, the power one has over one's possessions and one's self. This, in turn, legitimises contractual agreements as to how power should be used. According to early modern thinkers such as Hobbes or Grotius, we effectively 'trade in' the power we have to be in full possession of ourselves, in order to secure the protection from others attempting to take what is ours from us. In this way, our primordial 'natural' right becomes transferred into a civil or social right. The dividing line between the two, however, remains somewhat ambiguous. Ironically enough, with the advent of both the French and American Revolutions, this ambiguity only increases. The *Declaration des droits de l'homme*, for example, begins its preamble with a declaration that the rights of man are 'natural, inalienable and sacred'.[4] However, the rights it goes on to affirm are not only political and social, but also related to a highly specific political and social order.

For Hobbes and Grotius, who first proposed that society be based on a 'social contract', natural rights were not aligned with any particular organisation of society (this is precisely why they could be used by some parties to legally advocate for the colonisation of the New World at the expense of its native inhabitants, *and* by others to argue morally against it). But the French republic's 'Rights of Man' contain an irony which thinkers from Rousseau in the eighteenth century to Derrida in the twenty-first have commented upon. The rights of man are the rights of the individual. But these rights only make sense within the context of a civil society – after all, it would make no sense for someone to possess the right to be 'presumed innocent until judged guilty' (Article 9), unless they were already part of a judicial system which goes beyond their own individual existence. What this means, by corollary, is that one has no natural rights outside of society; because these are *only* guaranteed by the Declaration which, itself, presumes a society. In short: the individual only maintains their right to be an individual from within an established society. The idea of a natural right becomes inextricable from the notion of a social contract.

One effect of this in practical terms, which frequently comes to light in the aftermath of terrorist attacks within Western countries, is the limits of using human rights to defend civil liberties from heightened counter-terrorism measures. While human rights remain the legal basis to challenge government intrusion into the lives of individuals – keeping data on minority groups, tracking movements, and denying access to certain service provisions – the rights guaranteed are in fact the *same* rights that such terrorist activity threatens. This means that human rights struggle to balance the two senses of self-preservation that their history contains: self-preservation from the state, and self-preservation from those outside of the state. Hence, there is a clear knock-on effect of this regarding the extent to which an individual is at liberty to challenge the society they live within. As Pagden argues, following the *Declaration des droits de l'homme*:

> The rights of man were no longer those rights which could be held against society, or across differing societies. They were those which could only be held in society, and furthermore only in a society of a particular kind: republican, democratic, and representative. (Pagden 2003: 190)

This irony is continued when we consider the third ground of authority for such rights, which is freedom. This follows necessarily, as Joan Lockwood O'Donovan has noted. In a 'society whose only coherent public moral language is that of subjective rights', there can only be one universally respected right that all can agree on, and that is freedom 'from all externally imposed material and spiritual constraints on […] choice and self-determination' (Lockwood O'Donovan 1996: 63). But the problem with freedom is that it, too, presupposes its opposite. If freedom was naturally 'within' us, then we would not need a declaration of rights to uphold it. Instead, we require such declarations to ensure our freedom is maintained. This means that, as Stephen Webb points out, within social work and elsewhere such rights 'are effective only when there is a power to define and enforce them; they require an agent outside that is above their beneficiaries' (2009: 312).

When the UDHR was first drafted, one specific aim was to address this problem: rather than submitting the individual to the law of the nation, human rights allow the individual to challenge their own government or state authorities. Human rights are, in this sense, the ultimate defence of the individual against those who would take their freedom. However, the irony does not disappear. Firstly, the content of the UDHR – as we have seen in the criticisms made by Rawls and Cranston – remains political and social. Secondly, the core 'human' qualities it proposes continue to reflect the 'natural' rights of the early modern century European nations – the right to freedom, to property, and to contract. Thirdly, the UDHR maintains the problematic term of 'endowment', without a clear specification of which institution, body or entity this refers to. In this way, Pagden argues that the 'history of "human rights" may serve to remind us that if we wish to assert any belief in the universal we have to begin by declaring our willingness to assume, and to defend, at least some of the values of a highly specific way of life' (Pagden 2003: 173).

Thinking through Practice

In what cases would it be problematic if the ethics practised by social workers reflected a 'highly specific way of life'? Are there contexts where this would, in fact, be appropriate?

Third concern: are human rights appropriate to social work ethics?

But if human rights are, indeed, cultural artefacts masquerading as universal truths, then this is only half of the story. As Žižek outlines, there is also a:

crucial other half [which] consists in asking a more difficult, supplementary question: that of the emergence of the form of universality itself. How – in what specific historical conditions – does abstract universality become a 'fact of (social) life'? (Žižek 2005: 129)

In other words, why is the discourse of human rights so *persuasive* within practice itself? Given the previous discussions, how appropriate are human rights as a basis for social work values and ethics?

A key text in this debate is Stephen Webb's article 'Against Difference and Diversity in Social Work: The Case of Human Rights' (2009), and the subsequent discussion it generated. Webb identifies a particular approach to what he terms the 'right to difference', and the celebration of diversity it encourages within social work, as a corrupted and malign version of human rights discourse, that valorises the symbolism and language of rights over and above the contradictions it contains. Arguing against the likes of Ife and Witkin, then, Webb argues that 'if the bedrock of present-day social work ethics rests on the normative concept of human rights as worked through postmodern preoccupations with difference and diversity, then this is a morally bankrupt perspective' (2009: 308). In short, Webb's objection is that by focusing on difference – 'local, specific and culturally diverse movements, here, there and everywhere' (308) – social work loses sight of concrete political action, which involves identifying larger-scale, effective political movements. Social work ethics should be concerned, not with the maintenance of difference, but rather with the injustices and inequalities the celebration of difference might hide (309). If the discourse of human rights 'frequently represents aggregated individual free expression rather than collective action', then the universality promised by human rights is, in fact, only 'manifest in the relative difference enjoyed by diverse groups of oppressed peoples' (309).

Webb thus argues that it is social work's embracing of 'postmodern' ideals of difference, translated through the legal and political frameworks of human rights, which lead to a superficial and anti-political base for practice. 'If social work continues to endorse the postmodern conception of diversity and difference as the foundation for articulating a normative version of human rights', he contests, 'it is in fact contributing to a politics of symbolism over a politics of effects' (2009: 313). This point clearly targets those such as McDonald (2006) who, while accepting that human rights are necessarily idealistic, nevertheless offers a model for practice which allows for the service user to preserve their difference, their diversity, and by extension, their dignity. But Webb's assertion that this is merely a 'politics of symbolism' critiques this form of idealism: the distance between symbol and meaning carries with it a necessary projection into the future; a hesitation, a gap, a deferment, which becomes a space for idealistic dreams to mutate, rather than action occur.

In this claim, he is echoing the work of Alain Badiou in his short work *Ethics* (Webb 2009: 312). Badiou's target in this book, like Webb's, is the fuzziness of today's 'socially inflated recourse to ethics' (2001: 2). As a society, we know that ethics is *important* – we have ethics committees, ethical 'policies' and regulations – but we are not so clear on what ethics *is*, or who it is *for*. Explicitly, Badiou is hostile to the 'ethics of alterity', and 'identity politics': that is, the notion that specific identities – woman, black, homosexual and so on – are beneficial to the theorising of value. As his wider work reflects, Badiou's reformulation of ethics is an attempt to remove these differences from centre stage, and concentrate instead on what he sees as the more important concerns regarding the continued significance of truth, the concrete nature of possibility, and the importance of the 'event' to ethical proceedings.

In at least some sense, then, Badiou and Webb would seem to have no issue with Cranston's criticism of the second and third 'generations' of human rights, which effectively watered down the first generation. Likewise, Richard Hugman has argued that 'if human needs are regarded solely in terms of cultural difference, then claims to them as rights have insecure foundations, disconnected from their basis in a core of "what it is to be human" and partial to any given perspective' (Hugman 2013: 162). While cultural values are important, they are not core to rights-claims, which depend more on the common human needs of 'health and freedom'. However, both Cranston and Hugman maintain a rights-oriented approach to the question of ethics. For Badiou, as well as separating rights-claims from the 'postmodernists' (who are charged, by Webb, with advocating a naïve cultural relativism), we should also be wary of dogmatic liberalism and its rights-focused bases. Both liberals and postmodernists are, he argues, equally guilty of conservatism: the former of cementing difference, and thus causing the impossibility of ethical dialogue; the latter of obliterating difference altogether. But in between these two spaces – on the one hand, cultural relativism, and on the other hand, the dangers of reductive essentialism – there seems to be a space for a more authentic ethical activity. As Badiou argues:

> Rather than link the word to abstract categories (Man or Human, Right or Law, the Other...), it should be referred back to particular *situations*. Rather than reduce it to an aspect of pity for victims, it should become the enduring maxim of singular processes. Rather than make of it merely the province of conservatism with a good conscience, it should concern the destiny of *truths*, in the plural. (2001: 3)

Badiou's answer is to reappropriate truth as an ontological condition (as opposed to a social or discursive 'construction'). Truth retains its universalist authority, but universalism itself is not a collection of 'everything', but a sense of singular truth which is shared across all members of the world. 'Every universal presents itself not as a *regularisation* of the particular or of differences, but as a *singularity* that is subtracted from identitarian predicates' (Badiou and Žižek 2009: 30, my emphasis). In other words, what is universal must be thought of outside of any preconditions of culture or identity: they can only be singular 'events' which emerge without us having any framework or predicates to understand them as *anything other than* universal. Rights and laws can regulate identities and positions, but cannot provide 'an undivided subjective experience of absolute difference' (Badiou and Žižek 2009: 33). But what would? Badiou refers to four 'truth procedures' that can provide the basis of such events: love, art, science and politics. It is from these – rare, unexpected – moments, created through these procedures, that events emerge which are so undecideable that they bring into focus the singularity of the world: that 'the single world is precisely the place where an unlimited set of differences exist' (Badiou 2008: 63); that I can share in other people who 'exist as much as I do, even though they are not like me, they are different' (2008: 63). Badiou, then, as well as Webb (to an extent), does not reject the commonality or solidarity of ethics, but argues that this is always precariously close to its opposite: the celebration of difference as a way of removing any possible ethical ground between people, and instead an affirmation of the 'different worlds' they occupy.

Webb is certainly right to critique the platitudes of human rights discourse that often cover a lack of in-depth reflection on their moral grounding. At the same time, his alignment of such a discourse with 'postmodernism' is short-sighted. The enthusiasm of some social work theorists to typologise 'postmodernism' as a form of cultural relativism is clearly mistaken. But here it seems doubly so, given that much of the facile nature of human rights discourse is self-evidently *modern* (its emphasis on individual liberty, and resistance to the interference of others, for example) rather than reflecting anything like the work of thinkers such as Derrida, Deleuze or Baudrillard (see Gray and Webb 2013: 218), who have all critiqued European understandings of human rights as well as, incidentally, rejecting the term 'post-modern' to describe their work.

While this may be a minor point, it speaks to a broader problem with Webb's and Badiou's critique. Jim Jose quite rightly argues that Badiou 'collapses various lines of thought into all-encompassing generalisations' (Jose 2010: 247). As such, Badiou's argument 'is located within a particularly narrow philosophical milieu in which what he takes to be *the* ideology of human rights, or *the* concept of democracy, is assumed to be self-evident' (247). But he does not justify why he chooses to identify only one ideology and one concept. And, clearly, from our discussion so far, we can see that contestation is readily built-in to the very idea of what human rights may or may not be. Historically, the idea of a 'natural' right has served *both* imperialistic power *and* local resistance; it has *both* superseded political discussion *and* provided a ground for politics to take place, when all others had succumbed to violence. Omitting this tends to leave Badiou operating within 'straw man' arguments. He heavily focuses on specific thinkers (in the case of his *Ethics* book, this is mainly Emmanuel Levinas), but engaging with them as though their influence was universal. And, as Garrett notes, the same criticism can be made of Webb in a social work context, as 'the profession's "excitement" about "difference" is certainly not as prominent as [he] maintains; neither does it possess the hegemonic weight or doxic command that is suggested' (2013: 204–5).

Webb's argument should thus be seen as focused on the problem of identity politics (although it must be emphasised that the thinkers he commonly associates with this are rarely actual advocates). Seeing this as the fragmentation of social power that celebrates individual immanence at the expense of political change (see Gray and Webb 2013), he argues that an ethical approach must proceed from recognising the Same (rather than the Other), as it is only through this that the principles of equality and social justice can be restored to social work practice. In other words, simply enforcing the recognition of difference within ethical codes, as most professional social work bodies around the world do, as well as the IFSW, will not resolve this basic tension between the universality of ethical demands and the diversity of the people whom social work engages with. Furthermore, Webb argues, this fundamentally stymies any politically effective action social work can take. Ethics becomes an exercise in managing the risk of encountering others, rather than collaborating in social change.

For those respondents to Webb's article – in particular, Jim Jose (2010), Robert Imre (2010) and Peter Sohlberg (2009) – the problem could be said to be not the critique of human rights itself, but rather the same problem that we raised at the beginning of the chapter: if not human rights, *then what?* The framework which Badiou offers in the place of human rights is seen as an inconsistent and overly-polemical stance that is ultimately too generalising to be of use to advancing the discussion. Both Jose and Sohlberg criticise Webb for reducing 'universalism' and 'diversity' to two dichotomous entities. While Sohlberg simply refers back to the UDHR to 'demonstrate' how a balance is, in fact, achieved already (rather naively overlooking the history of the Declaration itself), Jose focuses instead on Webb's charge that celebrating diversity leads to depoliticising identity. This, he reminds us, is a complex political juncture between 'equal rights' as a force of social change (for example, universal suffrage), and 'equal rights' as a way of enforcing existing inequalities (for example, raising VAT on commonly bought food items, which disadvantages the poor). Rather, for Jose, it is precisely in that recognition of difference that a coherent social work ethics is most needed:

> Social work involves working with people who are usually, though not necessarily, located in positions of powerlessness. Hence, it follows that social workers are obliged both to recognise that difference and to take reasonable precautions with respect to their own conduct to ensure that they do not exploit or disempower those who seek (or are forced to seek) their assistance. And it is here that a concern for ethics is most pointed. (Jose 2010: 251)

Imre, meanwhile, agrees with Webb that the 'ethical turn' within social work seems to have had a negative effect on the political potential of social work, given that it often manifests itself as institutional regulation rather than group or individual empowerment. Instead, organisations are 'able to produce forms to complete in order to guarantee ethical behaviour from a strictly legalistic aspect, usually designed to protect the organisation from litigation, and this seems to stifle any real talk of ethics, and certainly works to stifle critique' (2010: 257). But, Imre notes, this does not in itself mean that the process is depoliticised. Ethics *itself* is not apolitical; it has rather become a medium through which organisations seek to depoliticise (or legitimise) their practices.

> **Thinking through Practice**
>
> When the BASW reviewed their code of ethics in 2011, they surveyed their membership for feedback on the existing wording. Several respondents noted the difficulty in upholding the ethical values of social work with the demand on resources and increasing work pressures (see McDonnell 2012: 27).
>
> To what extent is it important that social work ethics be thought of as regulatory or rule-based, given these criticisms? What are the benefits to practice, and what are the drawbacks? Conversely, how might a more open-ended and deep-rooted approach to ethics, such as Badiou suggests, fare?

Ethics and mediation: the *place* of rights?

It may seem strange that, for a chapter headed as 'ethics', it has taken this long to arrive at any substantial claims over the nature of social work ethics itself. But this is deliberately so. To discuss ethics in social work directly through the procedural or institutional 'rules' of practice is an approach which can lead to sidestepping the fundamental questions of an ethical code: how 'universal' are these? Should they always apply? What authority do they have over social work? Why are they here? It is precisely these questions that are brought to the fore by raising concerns over human rights as the base foundation of social work practice – even if, after all of this, we are happy to return to this foundation. Imre puts this well when he comments on the tension between universalism and diversity in human rights discourse that:

> Perhaps the real problem here is that social work, as a profession with a set of codes, practitioners who are very busy and people looking to do 'the right thing' or perform as a 'good social worker' in order to help people, need to open up to real diversity. In a practical sense, this is much more difficult than merely 'following the rules'. (Imre 2010: 258)

What does 'opening up to real diversity' mean here? This is far too big a question, of course – one that only a book-length treatment would do justice to – so in lieu of an answer, I want to close this chapter with three observations surrounding all of these concerns raised around the prevalence of human rights within social work ethics.

First, the question of human rights within social work seems to be not so much what human rights *are*, but in what situations and contexts, and as what kind of subjects or social actors, they emerge as *significant*. The history and philosophical underpinning of human rights are such that this will rarely be unambiguous – whether, for example, they are a legal ground, a moral directive, a guide for good practice, or something else. One of the problems with the more platitudinous invocations of human rights, which Webb rightly criticises, is that they are often superficial and empty references. But, following Imre's points, this might also suggest that the way in which human rights are invoked, or the place in which they sit within social work ethics, has more to do with organisational or professional standards, rather than the applied care or practice that the UDHR speaks to. Lena Dominelli identifies such a tension within the very question of what social work values are. Whereas the professional codes of ethics and frameworks for professional practice often attempt to identify clear and distinct value statements, Dominelli suggests that:

> ...reducing a set of values to one statement highlights the abstract nature of these values. When boiled down to one, it reaches levels of agreement and universality, which in practice become difficult to sustain in certain circumstances. If we are asked whether respecting the person is a key social work value, the question is cast in a decontextualized form and it is hard to imagine a social worker who would not overtly endorse it. However, posing the question in terms of practising values in context, the answers would be more nuanced and complex. (Dominelli 2002: 17)

Second, it is worth nothing that the discourse of human rights – whether critical or complementary – requires speaking 'big'. Whereas many practitioners may utilise the legal aspect of rights alone, the ontological basis of human rights is fundamentally moral and political as well. They can, and should, never be mere instruments of practice. When Peter Sohlberg notes that the structure of the UDHR means that 'social work would have to pay attention to the balance between universalism and difference rather than programmatically state preferences for one of the extremes' (2009: 318), this echoes a frustrated sense of searching for a *middle ground* within a discourse which is, at heart, *foundational*. This revisits an earlier question raised in the chapter: is social work not committed to a particular worldview, and the kind of 'highly specific way of life' that Pagden critiques human rights discourses for concealing? Is there a hint of confusion, in a comment such as Sohlberg's, between the technical ethos of practice – where balancing need and right is essential – and the norms and ideals which ground social work as a profession? Is one of the tensions between human rights and social work ethics, then, reflective of a more fundamental problem between the specific and the universal, between technical knowledge/capability and speculative knowledge/ethics, and between the local and the global?

Third, this involves a question of how we *access* rights, which is a question not simply about formal procedures in practice, but also the education of practitioners (e.g. how they become *aware* of what human rights are, when they can be referred to, why they are appropriate for particular modes of practice and so on), and how they are invoked – that is, discussed or represented – effectively. One of the problems with the 'textbook culture' that Webb criticises is that by sweeping over the inherent ambiguities of the UDHR, as well as the embedded multiplicity of texts, acts and bodies claiming the name of human rights, it can risk portraying misleadingly straightforward images of practice that muddy exactly how human rights are 'present' within interactions with service users. What the first two critiques of human rights show is that our access to them – as social workers, or philosophers, or both – is always regulated by social institutions and cultural traditions. This does not mean that there is no 'common humanity', or any shared norms or agreed norms. But it calls to attention that such commonality or shared agreements are always *mediated* in some way: by the ground they take place on, the roles we are called to play within them, the language we are necessitated to use, and so on. Often, it is such mediation that carries the effectiveness of our reflections and our discussions. Institutions and ideas operate within a hermeneutic circle, in this sense.

Thinking through Practice

How are human rights mediated within your practice? What effects might this mediation have on the way in which they affect the ethical basis of your work?

Notes

1 http://ifsw.org/policies/statement-of-ethical-principles/
2 See Hassan, 'Are Human Rights Compatible with Islam?', at http://www.religiousconsultation.org/hassan2.htm (accessed 04/12/2014)
3 It is important to note that the Western idea of 'morality' does not have an equivalent in Islamic thought, historically. Islamic 'ethics' are far more rooted in the law, which is (in turn) not an equivalent to the law in the sense often invoked by social workers during practice. So this paragraph is only making some rough claims that touch on a range of more complex discussions, that there is not the time to discuss here.
4 See https://chnm.gmu.edu/revolution/d/295/

References

American Anthropological Association, The Executive Board (1947). 'Statement on Human Rights.' *American Anthropologist*, 49, 4, 539–43.

An-Na'im, A. (ed.) (1995). *Human Rights in Cross-Cultural Perspectives: A Quest for Consensus*. Philadelphia, PA: University of Pennsylvania Press.

An-naim, A. and Deng, F. (eds.) (1990). *Human Rights in Africa: Cross-Cultural Perspectives*. Washington, DC: Brookings Institution Press.

Aquinas, T. (1954 [1256–1274]). *Selected Political Writings*. J. Dawson (trans.), A. D'Entreves (ed.). Oxford: Basil Blackwell.

Badiou, A. (2001). *Ethics: An Essay on the Understanding of Evil*. P. Hallward (trans.). London: Verso.

—— (2008). *The Meaning of Sarkozy*. London: Verso.

Badiou, A. and Žižek, S. (2009). *Philosophy in the Present*. P. Thomas and A. Toscano (trans.). Cambridge: Polity.

Beitz, C. (2009). *The Idea of Human Rights*. Oxford: Oxford University Press.

Bielefeldt, H. (2000). '"Western" versus "Islamic" Human Rights Conceptions?: A Critique of Cultural Essentialism in the Discussion on Human Rights.' *Political Theory*, 28, 1, 90–121.

Cranston, M. (1973). *What are Human Rights?* London: Bodley Head.

Dalacoura, K. (2003). *Engagement or Coercion? Weighing Western Human Rights Policies Towards Turkey, Iran and Egypt.* London: The Royal Institute of International Affairs.

Dominelli, L. (2002). *Anti-Oppressive Social Work Theory and Practice.* Basingstoke: Palgrave Macmillan.

—— (2010) *Social Work in a Globalizing World.* Cambridge: Polity Press.

—— (2012). *Green Social Work: From Environmental Crises to Environmental Justice.* Cambridge: Polity Press.

Donnelly, J. (1982). 'Human Rights and Human Dignity: An Analytic Critique of Non-Western Human Rights Conceptions.' *American Political Science Review*, 76, 2, 303–16.

Dworkin, R. (2011). *Justice for Hedgehogs.* Cambridge, MA: Harvard University Press.

Evans, E., Howlett, S., Kremser, T., Simpson, J., Kayess, R. and Trollo, J. (2012). 'Service Development for Intellectual Disability Mental Health: A Human Rights Approach.' *Journal of Intellectual Disability Research*, 56, 11, 1098–109.

Forrest, R. (2014). 'The Implications of Adopting a Human Rights Approach to Recovery in Practice.' *Mental Health Practice*, 17, 8, 29–33.

Garrett, P. (2013). *Social Work and Social Theory.* Bristol: Policy Press.

George, S. (2003). 'Globalizing Rights?' In Gibney, M. (ed.), *Globalizing Rights.* Oxford: Oxford University Press, pp. 15–33.

Gray, M. and Webb, S. (2013) 'The Speculative Left and the New Politics of Social Work.' In Gray, M. and Webb, S. (eds.), *The New Politics of Social Work.* Basingstoke: Palgrave Macmillan, pp. 209–24.

Greenawalt, K. (1987). *Conflicts of Law and Morality.* Oxford: Oxford University Press.

Haug, E. (2005). 'Critical Reflections on the Emerging Discourse of International Social Work.' *International Social Work*, 48, 2, 126–35.

Hobbes, T. (2008 [1640]). *Human Nature and de Corpore.* Oxford: Oxford University Press.

Hugman, R. (2013). 'Rights-based International Social Work Practice.' In Gray, M. and Webb, S. (eds.), *The New Politics of Social Work.* Basingstoke: Palgrave MacMillan, pp.159–73.

Ife, J. (1997). *Rethinking Social Work: Towards Critical Practice.* London: Longman.

—— (2012). *Human Rights and Social Work.* Cambridge: Cambridge University Press.

Imre, R. (2010). 'Badiou and the Philosophy of Social Work: A Reply to Stephen Webb.' *International Journal of Social Welfare*, 19, 253–58.

Jose, J. (2010). 'Rethinking Social Work Ethics: What is the Real Question? Responding to Stephen Webb's "Against Difference and Diversity in Social Work".' *International Journal of Social Welfare*, 19, 246–52.

Lockwood O'Donovan, J. (1996). 'Historical Prolegomena to a Theological Review of "Human Rights".' *Studies in Christian Ethics*, 9, 2, 52–65.

MacIntyre, A. (1998). *A Brief History of Ethics.* London: Routledge.

Mawdudi, A. (1976). *Human Rights in Islam.* Leicester: Islamic Foundation.

McDonald, C. (2006). *Challenging Social Work: The Institutional Context of Practice.* Basingstoke: Palgrave Macmillan.

McDonnell, F. (2012). 'The Code Makers.' *Professional Social Work*, January, pp. 26–7.

Nickel, J. (2007). *Making Sense of Human Rights.* 2nd edn. Malden, MA: Blackwell Publishing.

Oliver, M. (1990). *The Politics of Disablement.* London: Macmillan.

Orend, B. (2003). *Human Rights: Concept and Context.* Peterborough, Ontario: Broadview Press.

Pagden, A. (2003). 'Human Rights, Natural Rights, and Europe's Imperial Legacy.' *Political Theory*, 31, 2, 171–99.

Rawls, J. (1971). *A Theory of Justice*. Cambridge, MA: Harvard University Press.

Reichert, E. (2011). 'Human Rights in Social Work: an Essential Basis.' *Journal of Comparative Social Welfare*, 27, 3, 207–20.

Sohlberg, P. (2009). 'Is there Nothing beyond Postmodernism and "the Theoretical Other"? The Need for Balancing Universalism and Diversity in Social Work.' *International Journal of Social Welfare*, 18, 3, 317–22.

Twining, W. (2006). 'Human Rights: Southern Voices – Francis Deng, Abdullahi An-Na'im, Yash Ghai and Upendra Baxi.' *Review of Constitutional Studies*, 11, 2, 203–79.

Webb, S. (2009). 'Against Difference and Diversity in Social Work: The Case of Human Rights.' *International Journal of Social Welfare*, 18, 307–16.

Witkin, S. (1998). 'Editorial: Human Rights and Social Work.' *Social Work*, 43, 3, 197–201.

Wronka, J. (1998). *Human Rights and Social Policy in the Twenty-First Century*. Lanham, MD: University Press of America.

Žižek, S. (2005). 'Against Human Rights.' *New Left Review*, 34, 115–31.

5
DOCUMENTS
The politics of writing

The role of paperwork

A cursory glance over social work literature will reveal a noticeable discrepancy. Given the raft of reports estimating how long social workers spend of their contracted hours on paperwork,[1] there is a distinct absence of discussion on the idea of texts and documentation itself – at least, relative to the ever-increasing stockpile of resources available on interpersonal communication, relational practices and other associated fields. Mark Hardy goes as far as to say that, in some specific contexts such as recording residential child care settings, documentation is 'at present almost wholly untheorized' (2014: 108). And perhaps there is a straightforward reason for this: Savaya comments that 'most social workers [...] view documentation as a bureaucratic imposition that has little relevance to their work, client needs, or service provision, or as a necessary evil that takes precious time from more pressing work' (Savaya 2010: 661; see Prince 1996).

Nevertheless, if it is an evil, it seems a necessary evil. Bodek describes seven key reasons for documentation in social work:

1. To document professional work;
2. To serve as the basis for organisation and continuity of care by the practitioner;
3. To serve as the basis for subsequent continuity of care by other practitioners;
4. To provide risk management (agency, worker, and client safety) and malpractice protection;
5. To comply with legal, regulatory and institutional requirements;
6. To facilitate quality assurance and utilisation; and
7. To facilitate coordination of professional (or interagency) efforts. (Bodek, n.d.: 2, cited in Staniforth and Larkin 2006: 13)

It is not difficult to notice that in this list there is little mention of the more 'embodied' aspects of practice. There is a notable lack of terms such as caring relationship, social deprivation, community development and so on. In this sense, documentation seems to sit at the edge of social work; both in terms of its necessity to social work 'proper', but also as it so often operates as a medium between other agencies and professions. Frequently, 'paperwork' is aligned – for obvious reasons – with the Weberian sociological concept of bureaucracy, and in turn with a particular 'technical' approach to social work practice. 'Doing the paperwork' often appears to be something at odds with doing the face-to-face relational work that has traditionally been presented as something that is closer to 'proper' social work. Zastrow writes of the 'highly depersonalised, emotionally detached systems that view every employee and every client as a tiny component of a large system' (2009: 84). Administration becomes associated – often not unfairly – with managerialist watchwords like 'risk aversion' or 'budget monitoring'. And it is easy – again, sometimes for very good reason – to fall into a dichotomy between technocratic pen-pushing on the one hand, and dynamic, person-centred or psychosocial practice on the other (as in, for example, Trevithick 2003; Shaw et al. 2009).

It is worth remembering that, initially at least, the purpose of 'recording' practice was to provide a ground for theory building: in the earliest social work literature, documentation referred to research and teaching (Reamer 2005: 325; Cumming et al. 2007: 239). It was with the influence of psychosocial approaches and their use of personal narratives as a form of assessment, however, that documentation became more ingrained as part of casework itself (Callaghan 1996). Here, documentation was argued to be 'a tool to capture the essence of client-practitioner contact while helping the practitioner better understand the client dynamics' (Leon and Pepe 2010: 363). From here, the role of documentation reflected the emphasis on practice itself: for task-centred work, for example, text was an instrument through which to capture the salient attitudes and behaviours within a determined situation. Approaches such as task-centred models, which required a demarcated 'context' within which the social worker could practise, utilised (implicitly or explicitly) practice documentation in order to establish what this context *was*. The rise of behavioural therapies in social work in the 1980s likewise involved a negotiation between the recording of changes in the service user's activities, and the accountability of treatment – whether set goals had been reached, or other measures for the success of the intervention. Reflective models (Schön 1987), meanwhile, used documents as a way of monitoring a social worker's own responses to service users. This tended to remain a role of paperwork within social work education rather than practice itself, however (Kagle and Kopels 2008), and documentation became more prominently associated with accountability of practice rather than skills development. In the 1990s, meanwhile, a shift in the focus of documentation, in part facilitated by technological innovations in the way case notes could be recorded and stored, saw a new role for paperwork: risk management. It was these changes that led, in the US, to issues surrounding the recording of practice to be included as part of the revised NASW *Code of Ethics*, in 1996 (Reamer 2005: 327).

There is an interweaving of texts and practice, then, throughout the history of the profession, that does not express any one *specific* way in which the two are situated in relation to each other. Of course, it may be an obvious category error to see writing about research and writing up case notes as identical forms of textual practice, but I would argue that the philosophical problem of how text and action relate remains pertinent for both. Indeed, while the relationship between text and practice has perhaps come to be dominated by the managerialist-technocratic models of social work (see Garrett 2013: 5), it does not remove the work of textuality more generally within all approaches to practice. Likewise, if textbooks on documentation often take a prescriptive or corrective approach regarding some fundamental ideas of 'good writing', 'good note-keeping', and so on (see, for example, Weisman and Zornado 2013), this should not occlude the deeper question of the extent to which writing is 'secondary', in some way, to practice: that is, the principle behind the prescription. This is not to say that either the increase in bureaucracy, or the need for good writing, is insignificant or unimportant, of course. Rather, *before* we assert the need for the accuracy, appropriateness and ethics of documentation – needs which are often dictated by the context of writing, such as a clinical record, or managed care-plans (see Kane 2001) – there seems to be space to ask broader questions about the fundamental basis of such needs that cross different contexts of practice.

> **Thinking through Practice**
>
> What kind of problems arise when documenting your own practice, in terms of deciding what is relevant, what is appropriate, and whether what you're writing is accurate or not? In other words, to what extent do you find the act of documentation a *contested* area of practice?

While Bodek's list above appears to emphasise facilitation, legality and general instrumentality, it also speaks of paperwork as a 'basis'. On the one hand, it would seem that this basis would be nothing more than a provider of certain tools for social work to happen. As a tool, it would also be something to be picked up, dropped and replaced without particularly affecting the agency or values of its user. On the other hand, though, what if we considered this 'basis' as something more like a *ground* to practice, rather than an instrument? When, for example, we see directives that 'good social work recording should document reflective practice and that social work practice should be documented' (Cumming *et al.* 2007: 246), is there more to say about the precise relationship between reflection and writing? In other words, what if we saw the issue of documentation and paperwork as opening a broader philosophical question regarding the relationship between, on the one hand, thinking, acting and relating to others, and on the other hand, writing, reading and documenting? Might this be one way to think of the mediation of rights we mentioned in the previous chapter?

If the hard-pressed and overworked social worker sees documentation as a restrictive claw around their practice, the likes of Jacques Derrida and Paul Ricoeur have suggested that it is indeed textual forms which shape our world; but these should be recognised as ambiguous and polyvalent. The rise in material culture studies, cultural and sociological hermeneutics and post-structuralist deconstruction across the last 40 years or so has all suggested that it is:

> no longer appropriate to ask what a text means, what it says, what is the structure of its interiority, how to interpret or decipher it. Instead, one must ask what it *does*, how it *connects* with other things… (Grosz 1994: 199)

While Grosz is here referring to literary texts, readers and audiences, it should be noted that the ways in which material information connects and relates, and allows visibility of some things and maintains the invisibility of others, is a general aspect of modernity and late modernity. In this sense, 'textuality' goes beyond the actual idea of a text as a book or piece of paper, and applies equally well to the 'e-turn' in social work (see Garrett 2005). Boris Groys adds:

> bureaucratic and technological documentation serves as the primary medium of modern biopolitics. The schedules, regulations, investigative reports, statistical surveys, and project outlines that comprise this kind of documentation generate new life constantly. (Groys 2010: 82)

The idea of documentation 'generating new life' clearly conflicts with the sense of bureaucratic technology as a tool of managerial surveillance found at one time in social work literature (see Hough 1994). It does chime, though – however unintentionally – with Cumming *et al.*'s description of how 'paperwork' is perhaps less estranged from practice than it may first appear: 'the vital nature of documentation is […] relevant and applicable to all social work recording, irrespective of the medium being a paper or an electronic medical record', they argue, because the absence of such recording procedures brings social workers, service users, families and organisations into the domain of risk. 'It is when risk intersects with issues of rights, responsibilities, accountabilities, and integrity that it enters the realm of ethics and takes on a new shape within a framework that is generally well understood by social workers' (Cumming *et al.* 2007: 240–1).

Interpellation, identity and bureaucracy

It should be clear that this chapter is not championing the increase in bureaucracy in late modern social services. Rather, I am interested in exploring a more fundamental point about how texts relate to how we understand anything at all; and, following from this, what the significance of 'paperwork' might be as a form of creating, challenging or perpetuating power relations within practice and the world at large. To do this, we need first to think about how speech, actions and identities are formed through and in relation to documents.

Louis Althusser (1971) used the term *interpellation* to describe the way that individuals are 'hailed' by the social situation they enter, and the ideology which dominates it. Althusser's own example of this is a policeman who hails a passer-by in the street with 'hey you there'. At this point, nearly everybody in the street may turn around, as they all recognise themselves within the call. As Judith Butler summarises: 'the passerby turns precisely to acquire a certain identity, one purchased, as it were, with the price of guilt' (1997: 25). They turn around because they presume the policeman is talking to them, although this also assumes there is a reason the policeman is hailing them in the first place – in other words, they only respond in the knowledge that they are doing or have done something 'wrong'. This serves as an illustration of how 'people are assigned an identity according to the way in which they are positioned as subjects in discourse. [...] We put a label on people and expect them to live out their lives according to it' (Schram 2000: 53).

In her study of hate speech in the context of the law, Butler (1997) argues that this articulates how individuals are brought into being by the norms and structures, which are not only verbal but also textual, tactile and material. The individual only becomes an individual-as-such – that is, an individual who matters in this particular social context – at the moment they are called, and respond to the call. In turn, this coming into being as a subject has already been framed by a governing structure of power – we recognise the policeman before we recognise ourselves, effectively – and this limits the extent to which we can 'be' anyone outside of those ideological structures. Thus Butler argues that not only are 'the terms by which we are recognised as human [...] socially articulated and changeable', but that 'the very terms that confer "humanness" on some individuals are those that deprive certain other individuals of achieving that status' (Butler 2004: 2). While the case of the policeman is used for illustrative purposes – obviously we exist in some sense before someone shouts at us in a street – the point is that we are always-already a subject, in this way, because society operates through rituals of interpellation where we act out calls and responses. Such rituals of interpellation are, for Althusser, 'the material existence of an ideological apparatus' (1971: 168). It is such apparatus that provides the calling, and the language, by which we respond and identify ourselves.

Butler notes that while Althusser tends to privilege the voice as the main orchestrator of interpellation, it is also the case that, 'the efficacy of written or reproduced language in the production of social effects and, in particular, the constitution of subjects' is still felt closely:

> The interpellative name may arrive without a speaker – on bureaucratic forms, the census, adoption papers, employment applications. Who utters such words? The bureaucratic and disciplinary diffusions of sovereign power produce a terrain of discursive power that operates without a subject, but that constitutes the subject in the course of its operation. This does not mean that there are no individuals who write and distribute the forms. It means only

that they are not the originators of the discourse they convey and that their intentions, however strong, are not finally what control the meaning of that discourse. (Butler 1997: 34)

Here, Butler suggests that social identity is formed not simply on interpersonal relations (as social psychology has done much to inform us of) but also on our material relations to texts, forms, processes and other verbal or physical engagements with social 'systems'. An assessment form shapes the service user before they have answered the first question. In this sense, Butler notes that 'the boundary of the body never fully belongs to me' (2010: 54); or, indeed, is it necessarily a 'body' of flesh and blood.

Whereas for Althusser interpellation is a form of ideological oppression, for Butler interpellation is *inaugurative* (1997: 33). It is creative, as 'no subject can emerge without being differentiated' (2010: 141). Butler is interested specifically in how our identity in relation to such systems is often formed in particular moments – moments where we recognise ourselves within that system – rather than larger-scale structural explanations of how individuals are shaped. Power, for Butler, is 'diffused' through such moments of engagement: ideological norms are impressed upon the range of ways we are able to respond to the hailing. For example, a form asks for a person's gender, and offers 'male' or 'female'; it thus limits that person's identity to only two possible answers, and two gender identities (something Butler challenged in her most famous work, *Gender Trouble* (1990)). Conversely, we may think that two gender identities are enough, simply because those are the only options ever presented to us. The point here is not to specify exactly how many there might be; it is to suggest that our engagement with documentary materials is often through call-and-response scenes where our answers shape our sense of self. At the same time, however:

> If the schemes of recognition that are available to us are those that 'undo' the person by conferring recognition, or 'undo' the person by withholding recognition, then recognition becomes a site of power by which the human is differentially produced. (Butler 2004: 2)

Thinking through Practice

When does interpellation occur in social work practice? To what extent do social workers 'hail' service users, and in what ways might that 'hailing' constitute a service user's subjective experience?

What's the difference between text and action?

Social workers are constantly in the position of both hailing and being hailed, and perhaps one of the main ways social work inaugurates identities – as someone in need, as a 'service user', as a particular type of category of case (adult, child, mental health, etc.) – is through documentation. Of course, documents are records of activity (e.g. degree transcripts that enable registration; registration documents that enable practice; criminal record checks that enable work; care plans that enable successful practice, etc.), and thus possess a descriptive aspect. But they also, Butler argues, hold a constitutive and inaugurative role as well, whereby the 'hailing' (of, for example, the adoption form) creates a subject who did not fully exist before such a hailing. This role is rooted in the *difference* between texts and documents, on the one hand, and our spoken interactions on the other:

1. *Documents create distance.* Documenting an event involves a *transformation*, which Paul Ricoeur terms 'distanciation'. This happens in the following ways:

    First: 'the event of saying is surpassed by the meaning of what is said' (Moore 1990: 94). Writing preserves the meaning of something which may only happen, in real time, as a passing instant. Hence, Staniforth and Larkin assert, 'the purpose of recording [in social work] is to clearly establish the content and nature of our contacts with our clients', but also 'to illuminate the reason for the various actions that have resulted' (2006: 19). The distance within writing adds meaning to the passing event, in this way.

    Second: the author's intention and the meaning of the text separate themselves within writing. Documentation is provided in the first instance because of the *absence* of the person who writes it. In Ricoeur's words, 'the text's career escapes the finite horizon lived by its author. What the text says now matters more than what the author meant to say' (1981: 201). Conversely, reading documents is a form of 'supplementation' (Schram 2000: 48; de Man 1986), whereby what is missing from the text is supplied by the reader (and the 'cultural reserves' that they draw on to make such a reading). Documents can never be autonomous, in this respect.

    Third: Spoken words are usually addressed to a specific audience. Writing may also be directed to a specific audience, but because writing becomes, in theory at least, an object that anyone can pick up and use, the specificity within a spoken conversation is removed. Writing can shape its audience – the language it uses, the places it's kept, etc. – but this cannot *in itself* prevent anybody reading it. Staniforth and Larkin comment that it is 'not only our colleagues who need to understand the reasons for our actions, but also our clients who may read their notes and other third parties who may have an interest – especially those who may need to address the recording through a legal prism' (2006: 19). Indeed, what makes texts *available* or *unavailable* is rarely an act of speech, but rather further layers of material culture: either legislation on confidentiality, or physical obstacles such as locked filing cabinets or password-protected files on a computer system.

Fourth: In a conversation, words form references to a shared situation between interlocutors. The text 'does not refer to the situation of its production, but to the world' (Moore 2004: 94). Interestingly, efforts to improve documentation practices in social work have been far more successful when involving 'open access' or 'client access' to their own files, than when only involving increased training for accuracy (Gelman 1992). In other words, it is the awareness of this fourth distanciation – that a written document moves beyond its production and into the world – which seems to result in the most careful record-keeping.

2. *Documents are finite.* Unlike our lived experience, there is a beginning and an end to a document. This does not mean that there is necessarily a beginning or ending to its meaning – just because I have written case notes does not mean a colleague will understand precisely what was meant, if I have used ambiguous wording, or even bad handwriting. Rather, it means that there is an inevitable 'cutting' point in the act of documentation where notes must come to an end, where one box or the other must be ticked, where questions must be answered. Documentation in this sense is shaped by virtue of its *finitude*, and it is, indeed, precisely from this that it becomes so useful for transferring key points of information swiftly and clearly across to different parties.

3. *Documents are both ordered, and ordering.* Documents become sites of power, in Butler's words, largely through the bureaucratic systems they flow within. Documentation is never simply a piece of paper, but a system of information flow, replete with registries, archives, and control points affecting its circulation and storage. Max Weber (1992) famously wrote of an 'iron cage' of bureaucracy, whereby the rational order promised by bureaucratic systems, based on principles of efficient and cost-effect transference of information, is inextricable from the legitimacy of modern professional knowledge. At the same time, as James Beniger argued (1986), the 'control' over production and work that information systems promise often gives way to a 'storage crisis': the technologies of controlling information invariably create more information rather than less.

4. *Documents are expressions of our symbolic processes.* Documents are produced through signs, which in turn interrelate with other signs – not simply words and writing, but images, objects, clothes etc. – to form particular social identities. What this means is that so long as documentation in social work is a central part of the classificatory systems we use to make sense of the world, then it is also a form of *representation*. And, as linguists such as Norman Fairclough argue, a founding feature of representation is its link to the carrying and construction of power: they 'do not just reflect or represent social entities and relations, they construct or "constitute" them; different discourses constitute key entities [...] in different ways, and position people in different ways as social subjects'. (*Fairclough 1992: 3–4*)

Note that there may appear to be a tension between Fook's social work-specific list of dichotomies, and the more general list, regarding where 'texts' fit in. For Derrida, perhaps the most powerful representation of the metaphysics of presence was the privileging of speech over texts, as a 'purer' form of communication. For Fook, however, there is a clear sense that 'practice' and 'lived experience' are subjected to 'theory' or 'technical knowledge' within particular organisational and institutional contexts. So, on the one hand, Derrida's suggestion is that the metaphysics of presence would prioritise social work 'proper' as what is immanent and in the flesh, at the expense of what is merely an instrumental reflection of it: textual, helpful, but not essential. On the other hand, Fook suggests that lived experience is often only made visible through the lens of orthodoxies dictated by governing models of thought – hence, the popular refrain of literature on social work documentation that 'if it's not written down, it didn't happen', remains truthful because of the way in which the flow and processing of information structure social care provision.

Perhaps, though, this is not such a dilemma. Whereas dichotomies can be seen as *exclusionary* practices (see Levin 2009: 3) – one term utterly subordinates the other – Derrida argues that these dichotomies cannot simply be reversed by re-valuing the lesser term as a stronger one. Rather than being a simple choice between 'technical knowledge' and 'lived experience', Derrida's deconstructive approach alerts us to us how the desire for access to what is 'real' translates into a favouring of certain *modes of thought* over others. The problem is not, then, whether the 'reality' or 'propriety' of social work lies in the spoken word or the written text. The problem is rather the claim that either of the two will affirm a 'truth' which is both *immediately knowable* and *fundamentally complete*. It is this metaphysical need that renders writing a secondary substitute for speech, and text a supplement for action.

It is also what often shapes our capacity to critique these relationships, as our responses will always struggle to remove themselves from such pre-determined oppositions. This effect can often be seen when more radical approaches to social work are proposed, such as the critical social work movement, and are met with an instant demand to be a 'grounded and *practically useful* radicalism' rather than being 'left at the level of aspiration' (Ferguson 2013: 119, my emphasis). This is not to say that Ferguson's requirement of critical social work to offer positive as well as negative accounts of practice is not unfounded. Obviously, ideas also require action. The problem is more to what extent the distinction between the two is being drawn upon a metaphysical dichotomy (i.e. between 'theory' and 'practice'), and how this can affect the forms of knowledge which we recognise as appropriate. For Derrida, the dominance of presence as a form of truth is maintained by structures of power governing our interpretations and writing practices. However, he argues that such dichotomies, and the structures around them, are always inherently unstable and illusory. His approach is to demonstrate how each claim to authority, truth or legitimacy 'deconstructed' itself owing to its inability to ever achieve the immediately knowable and fundamentally complete status it required. In this way, deconstructions are ways of interrogating the assumptions that bind certain cultural and social practices together, and to challenge their inevitability.

> **Thinking through Practice**
>
> Take a straightforward example: what does the term 'social work' mean? How would you define it?
>
> Clearly, its meaning is derived from associative and contrastive terms; which, in turn, are also given meaning from further terms, and so on. A cursory glance over any textbook will tell you things like it is a caring profession (which must then be defined in relation to non-caring professions), it is an agency for social change (which must then be defined in terms of 'agency', 'social' 'change'), and so on; or conversely, it is *not* simply care management, or the ways in which it is *unlike* probation, nursing, occupational therapy, etc. Little surprise that even the most decisive definitions of what social work is, such as the governing statement of the International Federation of Social Work, are still contested and open to discussion. There is no 'complete meaning' to the term. Even at one moment in one context, the meaning will be dependent on shifting referential sands beneath it.
>
> This does not mean that there is no such thing as social work (if it did, it would be late in the book to take note of this!). On the contrary, the very fact that there *is* a thing called social work depends on its meaning never being fully complete. Meaning is not 'fixed' above and beyond the means of its production, which in this case is the production of a way of defining social work; which in itself requires there to be things that aren't social work to make any sense.

One cannot have meaning without difference; and what seems to be opposite or secondary to a name, occupation, or any kind of form turns out to be essential to it (Derrida 1976: 214). This introduces a gap within the idea of an 'immediate' meaning, which Derrida terms *différance*: a play on the French terms 'to differ' and 'to defer'. If the difference between action and text, or speech and writing, marks out an opposition, then *différance* refers to the space which both allows such an opposition to emerge, while at the same time rendering a full opposition impossible. Any sense of the 'immediate' is, therefore, always mediated in some way. Our sense of there being an 'immediate meaning' is maintained, though, by dichotomies which suppress this difference: *here's* what it is, *there's* what it isn't. On the one hand, this is simply a matter of convenience — it is easier to refer to an identity than an endless play of difference. With each assertion of identity — between speech and writing, power and powerlessness, worker and client and so on — the play of difference is cut, suppressed. On the other hand, this raises the fundamental question: for whose convenience? On what authority do we accept such identities? And in what ways are the differences and exteriorities suppressed, or repressed? How do we draw the boundaries between meaning and non-meaning? Deconstruction thus raises the question of what boundaries it is necessary to assume and protect for certain practices to get underway.

As we have seen, texts are often figured within social work as a medium for carrying information, and a risky one at that (Cummings *et al.* 2005; Reamer 2005). But the basis of this risk – that a document could be mis-read, taken out of context, or never arrive – is also the fundamental *task* of the document, as it must exist in the absence of its author. This 'iterability', Derrida argues, is in fact the task of all language: 'that language must traverse space [...] is not an accidental trait but a mark of its origin' (Derrida 1976: 232); and 'the possibility of disengagement and citational graft which belongs to the structure of every mark, spoken or written, and which constitutes every mark in writing before and outside of every horizon of semio-linguistic communication' (1988: 12). In this way, texts are not replications of our relation to the 'real' world; rather, our relation to the real world works the same as a text. Hence, for Derrida, there is 'no "outside-text"' (1976: 158).[3]

For example: while we may look at the interpellative practice of documentation as forming a distinct part of the assessment process, social psychologists and structuralist anthropologists alike have also told us that even in our basic interactions with people – even when social workers introduce themselves at the beginning of a meeting, for example – we are relying on categories, schemas and types to make sense of the unfolding dialogue. But such categories and schemas are never conclusive or fixed: the fact that you can place a service user's response to your opening speech in one category – 'happy', 'willing', 'angry', etc. – entails that you could also place it in another (or else you would not be able to place it at all). There is nothing that inherently links their response to your categorisation; only a set of relations governing your reasons for choosing one category over another. The meaning is not fixed. Whereas for structuralists our interpersonal relations reflect deep-rooted socialised systems of meaning, poststructuralists (following Derrida) highlight the unstable way in which these systems, as relations of reference and meaning, hold together.

Another example: when social work documentation is framed as a cooperative activity, formed by multiple agencies and actors, it tends to over-simplify the unified nature of such a community. It depends upon the idea of a 'community immediately present to itself, without difference [...] where all members are within earshot' (Derrida 1976: 136). But such an idea of a 'shared community' of intentional actors remains idealised (as inter-professional educators have long noted – see Barr *et al.* 2005). Our very identification of an 'actor' or 'speaker', in such a situation, is only a *postponement* or *deferral* of the discourse from which they speak. It is a kind of provisional localisation where we focus on one set of possible meanings, at the expense of others. The clarity through which we identify such agencies 'derives from that which it excludes, that which is withdrawn, removed, outside of it' (1978: 21). Of course, such a localisation is enabled by the social structures that social work takes place within doing much of this withdrawing for us; but these, in turn, are established as meaningful to us by other localisations, and other deferrals of possible interpretation. Such a localisation is never secure – the challenge of service user voices and alternative paradigms of practice demonstrate as much – but neither is it meaningless. Instead, it sits somewhere between collapse and completion: it relies on the presence and force of an 'original meaning', but only in order to postpone the fulfilment of such a meaning. Communication is not constructed from intentional actors, but deferrals of *intertextuality* that help us to understand the 'context' of what is being said. However, contexts are just like texts: we can never 'understand' them in a self-present, total way (Derrida 1988: 70). And if this is all a little abstract at this point, it can be summarised well by Parton and O'Byrne's suggestion that within practice, 'seeking to *understand* the problem is [...] a futile endless game; far better to accept and use our joint *misunderstanding* to begin constructing ways of solving the problem'. This depends upon recognising the inherent misunderstanding at work in any act of understanding: 'rather than say "let me try to understand" we can say "let me try to misunderstand less." What the problem is *not* [...] leads us to think of exceptions to the problem, [which] help us to see possibilities for change' (Parton and O'Byrne 2000: 56, my emphasis).

The reversal of the relationship between text and action is not a victory for bureaucracy, then, but rather the opposite. Derrida critiques harshly the belief that texts, or even language, can carry transparent and uncontested meaning, in the way that is frequently demanded of 'paperwork'. Rather, deconstructive reading 'does not point out the flaws or weaknesses or stupidities of an author, but the *necessity* with which what he *does* see is systematically related to what he does *not* see' (Johnson 1981: xv). As Hummel comments dryly, this is 'bad news for the managers', but 'good news for the hopeful citizen'. Good news, 'because attempts to use language as an instrument for social control now can be seen to produce the spaces for saying something original. Control produces its own lacunae, blank slates, uncovered realities – opportunities for escape. [...] Language has no fixed origin or end' (Hummel 2014: 150). And this instability – the way in which meaning, communication and writing all presuppose the very things that they mean to overcome – results in hope. In this way, writing is itself a *pharmakon* – both a poison and a cure. In Hummel's words, 'writing, in trying to secure what we mean, simply suggests the presence of the opposite: the insecuring of meaning'. Or, in short: 'writing, the tool of control, evokes the antidote to control' (Hummel 2014: 153).

If you didn't write it down, did it ever happen?

The legalistic term 'if it isn't written, it didn't happen' is frequently cited in the more protectionist accounts of documentation in practice. And it is this interpretative paradigm that textuality is frequently framed by. Note-keeping protects the social worker from later allegations; theoretical texts protect the social worker within a knowledge-economy; the register of social workers protects the public from bad practice, and so on. Derrida's argument is slightly different, and can perhaps be cast more as: 'if it happened, there is writing'. Despite the seemingly 'abstract' nature of what he says, and the difficulty in articulating its 'application' owing to having 'more in common with literary criticism than with writing and talking in [for example] child guidance clinics' (Prince 1996: 8), it nevertheless alerts us to how our approach to textuality is based on an interweaving of writing processes, which creates our sense of the limits of context itself. Derrida's account of textuality is important for challenging the basic dichotomy driven between text and action at the level of practice. In this way, it widens the discussion surrounding documentation from 'risk' – which may almost inevitably lead to an alignment of textuality with top-down, legalist methods of managerialist control – to articulating the ambiguous interface between document and user.

At the same time there are, of course, reasonable objections to such a discussion taking place. Let me consider three here: first, that the claim that there is 'nothing outside of the text' is ridiculous; second, that there is a clear tension between the instability and ambiguity which Derrida seems to celebrate, and the rigidity of bureaucratic culture within the social work profession; and third, that deconstruction offers no decisive position or politics that would justify social workers' interest in it.

The first objection can be summarised neatly by quote from a televised debate between the postcolonial theorist Gayatri Chakravorty Spivak, and the cultural critic John Dunn. Dunn articulates what many feel about Derrida's arguments:

> The view that all there is is texts is an absurd view. You only have to hear it to hear that it's absurd [...]. The radical insistence on textuality isn't any [...] obvious help in thinking about any of the major practical problems that face human beings politically, economically, etc. (cited in Spivak 1990: 24–5)

Dunn actually makes two points here. First, he claims that an over-emphasis on texts makes no sense. Second, he implies that there is a division between ethical or political questions of 'practice', and hermeneutic or interpretative questions of the text. In short, deconstruction makes no *sense*, and is of no *use*.

The idea that 'all there is is texts' is absurd largely because it is not an argument that anybody has really made. Dunn has approached the point about textuality while maintaining a rigid division between the text (the object) and its context (its construction, reading and writing). In this sense, of course it is absurd to claim that everything is a text. But this is not the sense in which Derrida uses the idea of a text. While for the likes of Ricoeur (1981), the writing and reading of texts are fundamental metaphors for social action, Derrida argues that texts cannot be seen as such complete entities, even as metaphors. Once we recognise the difference at play in any claim to meaning, he argues that 'the text is no longer the snug air-tight inside of an interiority or an identity-to-itself [...] but rather a different placement of the effects of opening and closing' (Derrida 1981: 35–6). Writing is more of a woven texture than a document: an 'interlacing that weaves together the system of differences' (Derrida 1981: 165).

If this is the case, though, a second problem arises when the ambiguities of deconstruction meet the demands of professional practice. The work of Michael Kane, for example, highlights a fundamental tension for US social work students who, on the one hand, face a bureaucratic culture which 'is becoming an ever-more critical piece in the delivery of services provided by social workers' as part of the increase in 'managed care', which contributes to lower morale amongst staff (Kane 2001: 56). On the other hand, though, this conflicts directly with the approaches to social work being delivered in the classroom, which Kane *et al.* propose more often reflect empowerment theories, strength-based perspectives, and postmodernist perspectives. Thus, while 'students are learning strength-based perspectives in academic settings, the managed care organizations in which they are employed or completing internships authorize services based on client deficits and identified problems' (2002: 200). This presents a 'conundrum' for both the ethics and education of documentation in the context of managed care, as the educator still:

> has an obligation to prepare students to interact with managed care organizations. The TASK becomes one of synthesizing favored social work theories with the REALITIES of utilization reviewers and managed care organizations. Educators, practitioners and students initially need an awareness that the language of the managed care organization may not always be the preferred language of the profession. (Kane *et al.* 2002: 208)

The problem is that 'postmodernism' here is seen in terms of language per se, rather than the mediation of language (i.e. the textual interweaving of identity and power within the discussion). As such, Kane *et al.* end up repeating a familiar dichotomy between theory and practice, or 'task' and 'reality' (even capitalising them to emphasise how different they are). The authors go on to assert that the imbalance between the two is an issue of 'preferred language' (2002: 209), and can be tackled by, first, an 'intensified dialogue between field supervisors and university faculty', and second, Patricia Kelley's suggestion that practitioners must learn to 'talk in two voices' (1998: 437) if they are to understand both the perspectives of their service users, and the realities of managed care. But this response lacks the richness of the original ethical conundrums they pose. There are several questions left unanswered: how stable is this language? What are the structures, references and supplements that allow this language to be 'preferred'? Is there a language of 'preference' *in itself*? Both of Kane *et al.*'s suggestions depend on articulating how the 'preferred language' is established. Field supervisors and university faculty are both constituted by more than just a relationship with a student, or a relationship with each other; these positions are formed through interpellation, inauguration and structures of difference.

The key here is that Derrida is not advocating an endless play of difference, or an infinite trace of meaning. Rather, his work questions how we draw such boundaries in the first place, and how implicated our own practices are within these. In other words, it makes no sense to insist upon harsh distinctions between 'task' and 'reality', 'supervisor' and 'faculty' or even 'student' and 'social worker' *without* attending to the medium through which these roles are constituted, and how complete and self-enclosed such constitutions are. This does not mean the distinction does not appear; rather, the key is not to 'talk in two voices', but to articulate what is deferred, and what is different, in the construction of the 'voice' itself.

On this point, du Gay (2000) has forcefully argued that the criticisms levelled at the 'bureaucratic' mind-set are often based upon accounts of management that are far too over-simplified. Du Gay's target is philosophers such as Alasdair MacIntyre who label the bureaucratic ethos of modern society as 'anti-moral' or 'a-philosophical'. This is, du Gay argues, to create an unnecessary dichotomy that cannot be sustained except in the most polemical of writings. Instead, not only do the likes of MacIntyre present an over-romanticised idea of free and creative 'pre-modern' thought that opposes managerialism, they also ignore the complexity and creativity of bureaucratic language and procedures (2000: 28–33; 40–2). In many senses, the technocratic face of social work arises as a contradictory consequence of a culture which prominently values *both* a sense of 'real occupation' (a lived, embodied experience of a working role), *and* a need to know 'what is really happening' (a verifiable, documented and accessible record of events we take part in).

Thinking through Practice

Do you think that du Gay's point could apply to the criticisms of bureaucracy within practice that we have seen so far? On what grounds might it not?

The third objection related to the lack of a clear politics to Derrida's observations. While there is a clear sense in which both Derrida and Butler have been keen to highlight how power enforces certain identities and dichotomies, it is true that deconstruction offers no 'new' or 'alternative' framework. It is not so much a method, as something that happens in any effort to enforce oppositional identity. It is not then surprising, perhaps, that Healy (2005) notes social work has been traditionally slow to pick up on the 'poststructural' turn in the social sciences; and while a concern with language, and therefore documentation, as an interactive process of identity construction has been developed, it often still subordinates writing to a reflection of speech (see Prince 1996: 48, 102). If anything, social work has been surprisingly quick to condemn poststructuralism as defunct or 'exhausted' (see, for example, Garrett 2013: 50), perhaps for the very reason that it 'casts fundamental doubt on the humanist orientation of social work and refuses to offer any ideological alternative' (Harris 2001: 336). Sanford Schram argues that deconstruction can 'provide an opening for contextualising, narrating, and understanding the problems of welfare policy differently' (Schram 2000: 139); but this is predicated on there being a space in which such contextualising and understanding can take place – a space which deconstruction itself resists articulating.

Perhaps such a space does not have to necessarily be a full-blown 'poststructural social work', however (see Fawcett 1998; Harris 2001). Instead, perhaps Derrida's points on textuality simply serve to raise far more humble questions over how we draw the boundary between documentation and 'proper' social work. In their critique of the Common Assessment Framework (CAF) – a standard assessment tool for UK professionals working with children – White, Hall and Peckover (2009) argue that such forms place both a descriptive and interpretative demand on workers. The CAF is 'designed to be evidence-based, focused on needs and strengths, rather than "concerns". Narratives are designed out' (2009: 1203). But the researchers found that such a categorical approach 'ignores the interactional nature of communications' (1214), replete with the narratives and reflexivity which allow service user needs to be recognised. As a result, they discovered that 'form-completers are attending reflexively to the institutional purposes of the CAF', by 'using it to manage accountabilities and accomplish disposals in locally artful ways' (1212). Drawing on the work of Michel Serres, who shares much of his approach with that of Derrida (see Assad 1999), they conclude:

> communications within a system are embedded in a range of interpretive dichotomies, signal/non-signal, information/noise and pattern/randomness (Serres, 2007), each with semi-permeable boundaries. One reader/hearer may find information where another can find only noise. […] [T]his makes a common language not only unattainable, but undesirable, because 'noise' has the potential to bring vitality and the hope of fresh patterns. The CAF may not provide a common language, because of the permeable interpretive interface. But, we should perhaps celebrate this 'failure', because the alternative has the potential to become a relatively 'noise-free' bank of cant phrases. (White *et al.* 2009: 1214)

This is not an example of 'deconstruction in action' – far from it – but rather points to the ways in which textuality underlies not only the interpellative nature of social work practice, but also its narrative elements which help social workers and their clients 'make sense' of the situation at hand. If bureaucracy can shape practice, then practice can unpick the weave of such documents in order to explore what is marginalised within its demands. In a different paper, White *et al.* make an impassioned plea for 'practice-near' research in order to shape systems and technologies for reforming practice (2009: 407). Their ethnographic study of social workers in the UK using the Integrated Children's System (ICS) highlights how top-down, centralised bureaucratic systems that insist on self-enclosed performance targets were producing both unsafe practice (such as a dangerous backlog of cases) and resistance from social workers and service users alike (409). But while, on the one hand, they draw a clear opposition between the time social workers spend 'entering data, mechanistically following bureaucratic procedures' and its diminishing effect on 'the time available for careful investigation of individual family circumstances, and engaging directly with real people and their lives' (2009: 409), this is not to simply assert the dominance of one over the other. Rather, we can see their findings as speaking to the way in which the *suspension of intertextuality* affects practice. Hence, White *et al.* critique the design of the ICS for not recognising either the ways in which service users interpreted its processes, or the resistance from social workers themselves: in other words, to use the language of deconstruction, for closing down the intertextual practices which were necessary for its successful completion.

Derrida's account shows how instabilities within the systems of documentation processes are inherent to any form of writing. Texts are never simply 'instrumental', and are never simply 'innocent'. They cannot be equated to 'discourse', in the quasi-Foucauldian manner that has tended to dominate the social scientific influence on social work theory. For all the straw man arguments that have been levelled against the deconstructive focus on textuality, it remains the case that texts are central to what Bourdieu identifies as the key for any struggle for meaning in the social world: what is at stake, he argues, 'is power over the classificatory schemes and systems which are the basis for the representation of groups and therefore of their mobilization and demobilization' (Bourdieu 1984: 479).

Of course, such classificatory schemes do not come down to documents alone, and any analysis will also involve a myriad of other areas: power, identity, discourse, territorialisation, and so on. And of course, we may want to limit the discussion of documentation in social work to clear bureaucratic texts such as 'caseload management schemes, child protection registers and statements of special educational needs' (Prince 1996: 10). But when we think of 'practice guidelines' solely in terms of their verbosity rather than the medium through which they appear to us, and if we think of 'training' in terms of the end practice, rather than the interplay of documentary systems by which training is formulated, ordered and recorded, then even if we are not happy with Derrida's insistence that there is nothing outside the text, the unbalanced relationship between text and action nevertheless requires philosophical justification.

Notes

1   For example, in a recent report for the Northern Ireland Association of Social Workers, polemically entitled *Social Work not Paperwork*, a survey of social workers found 96 per cent of participants highlighted report writing, and 90 per cent recording in client files, as a specific difficulty that impacted on their ability to spend time in face-to-face work with clients (NIASW 2012: 6).
2   Any claim over the entire history of 'Western philosophy' is, of course, likely to be polemical and overly broad. This is in part because the singularity of the 'tradition' of Western philosophy is more of an amalgamation of different approaches than one unbroken line of thought (indeed, Derrida contested this idea). Within this amalgamation, however, the *dominant* strands of thinking – those which commandeer what counts as 'making sense'; rationalism, empiricism, positivism and so on – have expressed these dichotomies, with consequences that are not simply undone by finding small exceptions to the rule (any more than one case of neglectful service provision renders the concept of social care redundant).
3   This is the literal translation of Derrida's infamous statement *il n'y a pas de hors-texte*. It has more commonly been translated as 'there is nothing outside of the text', which is what leads critics such as Dunn (later on in this chapter) to falsely claim that Derrida is denying 'reality' by claiming that everything is a text.

References

Althusser, L. (1971). *Lenin and Philosophy and Other Essays*. B. Brewster (trans.). New York: Monthly Review Press.
Assad, M. (1999). *Reading with Michel Serres: An Encounter with Time*. New York: SUNY Press.
Barr, H., Koppel, I., Reeves, S., Hammick, M. and Freeth, D. (2005). *Effective Interprofessional Education: Argument, Assumption and Evidence*. Oxford: Blackwell Publishing.
Beniger, J. (1986). *The Control Revolution: Technological and Economic Origins of the Information Society*. Harvard, MA: Harvard University Press.
Bourdieu, P. (1984). *Distinction: A Social Critique of the Judgement of Taste*. R. Nice (trans.). Harvard, MA: Harvard University Press.
Butler, J. (1990). *Gender Trouble*. London: Routledge.
—— (1997). *Excitable Speech*. London: Routledge.
—— (2004). *Undoing Gender*. London: Routledge.
—— (2010). *Frames of War: When is Life Grievable?* London: Verso.
Callahan, J. (1996). 'Documentation of client dangerousness in a managed care environment.' *Health and Social Work*, 21, 202–8.
Cumming, S., Fitzpatrick, E., McAuliffe, D., McKain, S., Martin, C. and Tonge, A. (2007). 'Raising the Titanic: Rescuing Social Work Documentation from the Sea of Ethical Risk.' *Australian Social Work*, 60, 2, 239–57.
De Man, P. (1986). *Resistance to Theory*. Minneapolis, MN: University of Minnesota Press.
Derrida, J. (1976). *Of Grammatology*. G.C. Spivak (trans.). Baltimore, MD: Johns Hopkins University Press.
—— (1981). *Dissemination*. B. Johnson (trans.). Chicago, IL: University of Chicago. Press.
—— (1988). *Limited Inc*. S. Weber and J. Mehlman (trans.). Evanston, IL: Northwestern University Press.
Du Gay, P. (2000). *In Praise of Bureaucracy: Weber – Organization – Ethics*. London: Sage.
Fairclough, N. (1992). *Discourse and Social Change*. Cambridge: Polity.
Fawcett, B. (1998). 'Disability and Social Work: Applications from Poststructuralism, Postmodernism and Feminism.' *British Journal of Social Work*, 28, 2, 263–77.
Ferguson, H. (2013). 'Critical Best Practice.' In Gray, M. and Webb, S. (eds.) *The New Politics of Social Work*. Basingstoke: Palgrave Macmillan, pp. 116–27.
Ferguson, I. and Woodward, R. (2009). *Radical Social Work in Practice: Making a Difference*. Bristol: Policy Press.
Fook, J. (2002). *Social Work: Critical Theory and Practice*. London: Sage.
Garrett, P. (2005). 'Social Work's "Electronic Turn": Notes on the Deployment of Information and Communication Technologies in Social Work with Children and Families.' *Critical Social Policy*, 25, 4, 529–53.
Garrett, P. (2013). 'Mapping the Theoretical and Political Terrain of Social Work.' In Gray, M. and Webb, S. (eds.), *The New Politics of Social Work*. Basingstoke: Palgrave Macmillan, pp. 44–62.
Gelman, S. (1992). 'Risk Management through Client Access to Case Records.' *Social Work*. 37, 1, 73–9.
Grosz, E. (1994). 'A Thousand Tiny Sexes: Feminism and Rhizomatics.' In Boundas, C. and Olkowski, D. (eds.), *Gilles Deleuze and the Theater of Philosophy*. London: Routledge, pp. 187–210.
Groys, B. (2010). *Going Public*. New York: Steinberg Press.
Hardy, M. (2014). 'Shift Recording in Residential Child Care: Purposes, Issues and Implications for Policy and Practise.' *Surveillance & Society* 12, 1, 108–23.

Harris, P. (2001). 'Towards a Critical Post-structuralism.' *Social Work Education*, 20, 3, 335–50.
Healy, K. (1999). 'Power and Activist Social Work.' In Pease, B. and Fook, J. (eds), *Transforming Social Work Practice*. London: Routledge, pp. 115–34.
—— (2005). *Social Work Theories in Context: Creating Frameworks for Practice*. Basingstoke: Palgrave Macmillan.
Hough, G. (1994). 'Post-Industrial Work? The Use of Information Technology in the Restructuring of State Social Work.' In Ife, J., Leitman, S. and Murphy, P. (eds.), *Advances in Social Work and Welfare Education*. National Conference of the Australian Association for Social Work and Welfare Education, pp. 56–62.
Hummel, R. (2014). *The Bureaucratic Experience: The Post-Modern Challenge*. London: Routledge.
Johnson, B. (1981). 'Translator's Introduction.' In Derrida, J. (ed.), *Dissemination*. Chicago, IL: University of Chicago Press, pp. vii-xxxiii.
Kagle, J. D. and Kopels, S. (2008). *Social Work Records*. 3rd edn. Long Grove, IL: Waveland Press.
Kane, M. (2001). 'Are Social Work Students Prepared for Documentation and Liability in Managed Care Environments?' *The Clinical Supervisor*, 20, 2, 55–65.
Kane, M., Houston-Vega, M. and Nuehring, E. (2002). 'Documentation in Managed Care: Challenges for Social Work Education.' *Journal of Teaching in Social Work*, 22, 1, 199–212.
Kelley, P. (1998). 'Postmodern approaches: Education for a Managed Care Environment.' In Schamess, G. and Lightburn, A. (eds.), *Humane Managed Care?* Washington, DC: NASW Press, pp. 430–41.
Leon, A. and Pepe, J. (2010). 'Utilizing a Required Documentation Course to Improve the Recording Skills of Undergraduate Social Work Students.' *Journal of Social Service Research*. 36, 4, 362–76.
Levin, I. (2009). 'Discourses Within and About Social Work.' *Journal of Comparative Social Work*, 1, 1–18.
Moore, H. (1990). 'Paul Ricoeur: Action, Meaning, and Text.' In Tilley, C. (ed.), *Reading Material Culture*. Oxford: Basil Blackwell, pp. 85–120.
Northern Ireland Association of Social Workers (2012). 'Social Work not Paperwork: Cutting Bureaucracy in Childcare Social Work.' Available at http://cdn.basw.co.uk/upload/basw_32936-10.pdf (last accessed 22/01/2015).
Parton, N. and O'Byrne, P. (2000). *Constructive Social Work: Towards a New Practice*. Basingstoke: Palgrave Macmillan.
Prince, K. (1996). *Boring Records? Communication, Speech and Writing in Social Work*. London: Jessica Kingsley Publishers.
Reamer, F. G. (2005). 'Documentation in Social Work: Evolving Ethical and Risk-Management Standards.' *Social Work*, 50, 4, 325–34.
Ricoeur, P. (1981). *Hermeneutics and the Human Sciences*. J.B. Thompson (trans.). Cambridge: Cambridge University Press.
Savaya, R. (2010) 'Enhancing Student Awareness of the Importance of Full and Accurate Documentation in Social Work Practice.' *Social Work Education*, 29, 6, 6060–9.
Schön, D. (1987). *Educating the Reflective Practitioner: Toward a New Design for Teaching and Learning in the Professions*. Oxford: Wiley Blackwell.
Schram, S. (2000). *After Welfare: The Culture of Postindustrial Social Policy*. New York: New York University Press.
Serres, M. (2007). *Parasite*. Minneapolis, MN: University of Minnesota Press.
Shaw, I., Bell, M., Sinclair, I., Sloper, P., Mitchell, W., Dyson, P., Clayden, J. and Rafferty, J. (2009). 'An Exemplary Scheme? An Evaluation of the Integrated Children's System.' *British Journal of Social Work*, 39, 4, 613–26.

Spivak, G. C. (1990). *The Post-Colonial Critic: Interviews, Strategies, Dialogues*. London: Routledge.

Staniforth, B. and Larkin, R. (2006). 'Documentation in Social Work: Remembering our ABCs.' *Social Work Review*, 18, 3, 13–20.

Trevithick, P. (2003) 'Effective relationship-based practice: a theoretical exploration.' *Journal of Social Work Practice*, 17, 2, 173–86.

Vattimo, G. and Zabala, S. (2011). *Hermeneutic Communism: From Heidegger to Marx*. New York: Columbia University Press.

Weber, M. (1992 [1904]). *The Protestant Ethic and the Spirit of Capitalism*. T. Parsons (trans.). London: Routledge.

Weisman, D. and Zornado, J. (2013). *Professional Writing for Social Work Practice*. New York: Springer.

White, S., Hall, C. and Peckover, S. (2009). 'The Descriptive Tyranny of the Common Assessment Framework: Technologies of Categorization and Professional Practice in Child Welfare.' *British Journal of Social Work*, 39, 1197–217.

White, S., Broadhurst, K., Wastell, D., Peckover, S., Hall, C. and Pithouse, A. (2009). 'Whither Practice-Near Research in the Modernization Programme? Policy Blunders in Children's Services.' *Journal of Social Work Practice*, 23, 4, 401–11.

Zastrow, C. (2009). *Introduction to Social Work and Social Welfare: Empowering People*. Belmont, CA: Cengage Learning.

6
SELF

Who am I, and what do I actually do?

The self in history

Philosophical questions of the self traditionally concern the emergence and persistence of identity: how do I know who I am, and how do I know that I am the same 'I' over the course of time? How do I account for the changes that happen to my body, beliefs and behaviours while maintaining a sense of who I am? In this sense, such questions underly the subsequent debates over the practical, political and ideological stances that social work theory and education have engaged in over the years. While social work education has long advocated the 'use of self' within reflective learning (Pallisera *et al.* 2013), the question of exactly what *constitutes* this self reflects a core contestation over the purpose and value of social work practice itself. Different conceptions of selfhood have driven the disposition of practice. The development of a service user's 'character' was, for example, fundamental to the moral idealism of the Charity Organisation Societies of the late nineteenth century. The question of self was intrinsic to the move, in the interwar period, away from biomedical accounts of 'health' to psychoanalytic approaches in clinical social work, where the self was understood as holding hidden depths that the practitioner could unearth. It was likewise embedded within the therapeutic turn of the psychodynamic models of social work within the 1970s, where 'self-actualisation' became a key mantra. And in contemporary practice, contrasting accounts of the self drive both the neoliberal 'personalisation' agenda (see Pierson 2011: 199–203), and the person-centred debate on the 'politics of recognition' that has recently emigrated from political philosophy to social work theory (see Marthinsen and Skjefstad 2011). It is not surprising, then, that the question of self-identity within social work has historically sat in tension: whether between those answers embedded within models of 'casework' and their psychological or therapeutic emphases (see Greene 2008), and the 'structural' understandings of identity that require more substantive social change put forward by radical and Marxist social work perspectives (see Payne 2005); or between what Parton and O'Byrne distinguish as the 'technical-rational' approach to practice, which emphasises scientific, evidence-based and outcome-focused work, and a 'practical-moral' approach that recognises the tacit and implicit knowledge of practitioners which recognises uncertainty and doubt at the core of practice (2000: 30-1). These are not simply different areas of focus, but rather different narratives of what social work is *for* at the most fundamental of levels: 'these debates are not just about ideology; rather, they support certain ways of knowing and behaving while discouraging others' (Daniel and Quirros 2010: 283)

The philosophical concern, then, is with that first point: the meaning of the 'I' that begins all of the debates above. Of course, this question may seem so obvious and immediate – after all, what could be more intimate than our own self? – that we move immediately to the epistemological and moral questions that follow. But it is precisely the philosophical question of the nature of the self that forms the ground – and thus shapes the limits and possibilities – for those epistemological and moral questions. Indeed, in many senses the modern era begins with René Descartes' argument that *cogito ergo sum* – 'I think, therefore I am' – and the discovery of a *specific* sense of self as rational and objective. In one of the most famous opening lines to a work of philosophy, Descartes begins his meditation by noting 'the large number of falsehoods that I had accepted as true in my childhood, and [...] the highly doubtful nature of the whole edifice that I had subsequently based on them' (1986: 12). He therefore sets out to determine what he can know *for certain*, by doubting anything that could possibly be doubted: the traditions he has learned from (which could be misleading), his own senses (as they have deceived him before), the 'real' world around him (which he could be dreaming), and so on until he realises the only thing that he cannot possibly doubt – and therefore the only thing he can know for certain – is that there is something actually doing the doubting. From this point on, this doubting thing – the Cartesian self – is the foundation of the certain knowledge with which he can refurnish the world. In doing so, Descartes establishes a standard principle for modernity: the emphasis on rational, objective and certain knowledge, knowable to *me*. This dualism between subject and the object – whereby knowledge, even of the self, must be an object for the rational appraisal of the subject – is what separates modern philosophy from its humanist predecessor, where there was far less distinction between science, art and ethics (Lash 1999: 42). The errors of Descartes' childhood are, of course, analogical to the development of society itself. The increasing redundancy of previously dominant ideas about the world – that the Sun orbited the Earth, for example – and the violent and bloody disagreements over the nature of the 'divine' or 'natural' laws that ravaged the fifteenth and sixteenth centuries, prompted a need for new foundations of knowledge. The turn to the self in Descartes' *Meditations* was thus reflective of the broader turn within European society, away from knowledge that had previously been guaranteed by a social and religious order beyond human intervention, and towards a more immediate and immanent sense of certainty guaranteed by the individual. And whether this individual was formed through Descartes' rationalist philosophy, the empiricist philosophy of the likes of John Locke or David Hume, or the idealist philosophy of Kant, the dominant currents of modern thinking retained at their core a self who observed, assessed and decided upon the nature of the reality around them: and in this way, the 'practical arts of the human sciences were derived from their desire to make a new man [*sic*] for the emerging social order' (Schram 2000: 64; see Foucault 1984).

While there are any number of routes into thinking about the nature of the self in between social work and philosophy, in this chapter I want to focus on one particular discussion based on Charles Taylor's critique of the dominant model of the modern self which I have briefly sketched out above, and its relation to the self within social work education. The demands of a self 'in training' within the context of social work pose, I think, some intriguing questions for this particular debate within the philosophy of identity to answer.

Knowing where I stand: what is 'the self' in social work education?

The mass transformations of modernity – industrialisation, urbanisation, globalisation, neo-liberalism; the collapse of traditional moral authorities and the redundancy of 'metanarratives' (Lyotard 1984) – affect intimate changes in our self-identity. As such:

> [T]he question is often spontaneously phrased by people in the form: Who am I? But this can't necessarily be answered by giving name and genealogy. What does answer this question for us is an understanding of what is of crucial importance to us. To know who I am is a species of *knowing where I stand*. My identity is defined by the commitments and identifications which provide the frame or horizon within which I can try to determine from case to case what is good, or valuable, or what ought to be done, or what I endorse or oppose. In other words, it is the horizon within which I am capable of taking a stand. (Taylor 1989: 27, my emphasis)

In other words, the self cannot be understood in simple quantitative terms, by looking back at where we've come from. Instead, echoing Gadamer (see Chapter 1), Taylor argues that the self is 'the horizon within which I am capable of taking a stand': I am always projecting forward, valuing and judging the best route forward. Initially, at least, this may seem relatively straightforward. A prospective student is asked at interview why they want to be a social worker, and they reply: I want to make a difference. I want to help. I think I would be good at it. 'Ideally,' Basham and Buchanan argue, 'students who pursue social work education should be well suited to advancing the profession's foundational goal of bettering the human condition' (2009: 187).

So why might 'knowing where I stand' be a problem in the first place? If students begin with a sense of what Taylor describes as 'what is good, or valuable, or what ought to be done', then the translation of this into an embodied sense of self is a harder task. Historically, social work theorists have struggled to locate a clear sense of what kind of 'self', philosophically speaking, sits within social work education. Back in 1980, for example, Brewer and Lait launched a stinging criticism of social work precisely for its overly-broad range of definitions, functions, standards and training (1980: 8). More recently Earls Larrison and Korr have noted, from a very different perspective, that the notion of the 'professional self' is left implicit rather than explicit within the North American proficiencies: 'the current standards provide limited educational emphasis, direction, or necessity for the specific application, use, and development of the *professional self* within the structure or curriculum of social work programs' (2013: 204, my emphasis). The case is made from both ends of the continuum: for Earl Larrisson and Korr, the answer is to embed the identity of the professional self within the practical wisdom of the profession. Brewer and Lait, meanwhile, argued that a reduction of curriculum was necessary, along with an abandonment of the idea of social work being a profession at all.

For our purposes, we can focus on a particular tension within the self implied by certain professional standards. In the United States, the Council on Social Work Education's (CSWE) Educational Policy and Accreditation Standards (EPAS) opens with a declaration that social work is guided, amongst other things, by 'a knowledge based on scientific inquiry'. Further on, Educational Policy 2.1.3 on the application of critical thinking states that social work knowledge is built upon an understanding of 'the principles of logic, scientific inquiry, and reasoned discernment. […] Social workers distinguish, appraise, and integrate multiple sources of knowledge, including research-based knowledge and practice wisdom (CSWE 2008: 4). In the United Kingdom, domain six of the College of Social Work's (TCSW) Professional Capabilities Framework (PCF) shares virtually identical wording. Likewise, the fifth domain of the PCF on 'Knowledge' states that social workers 'understand psychological, social, cultural, spiritual and physical influences on people; human development throughout the life span and the legal framework for practice'; which is applied 'in their work with individuals, families and communities.' (College of Social Work 2012: 2); whereas the EPAS 2.1.7 affirms that 'social workers apply theories and knowledge from the liberal arts to understand biological, social, cultural, psychological, and spiritual development' (2008: 6). Requirements such as these, aimed at consolidating the identity of the social worker from training onwards, in fact open up a number of different ways in which the self can be thought of.

There are, of course, a myriad of historical, political and pedagogical reasons as to why these standards appear in their current form (see Reisch and Andrews 2002; Jennissen and Lundy 2011; Dulmus and Sowers 2012). But in terms of the question of self, we are interested here in two points in particular.

Firstly, it is obviously simplistic to imagine that psychology, society and spirituality utilise the same concept of what the self is. Within each area we will find an entire range of competing ideas as to what constitutes a self, and to what purpose: for example, what Parton and O'Byrne refer to as the 'psy complex', which links psychoanalysis, psychology and psychotherapy, situates human qualities 'as measurable and calculable and thereby [...] [capable of being] changed, improved and rehabilitated' (2000: 38). Spiritual development, however, speaks a different language: and one that, as Peter Edwards notes, can often be seen as at odds with the social and material focus of the social work role (2002: 78–9). It is a similar problem when we try and think of the self that is studied and discussed in the liberal arts as identical to the self under the microscope of biomedical science. In each case, it could be argued that these are merely facets of the same self – that is, I may write a poem about how my emotions feel to me, and do a brain scan to see what my emotions do to me, but it is the same 'thing' that is being examined in both – but that would overlook just how different particular theories (particularly in psychology and sociology) can develop in utterly contrasting ways, based on their fundamental philosophical position on what the self is. What the EPAS and the PCF reflect, then, is less a coherent sense of self, and more of what Camilleri notes as the longstanding dispute over whether social work is a 'science' or an 'art' (1999: 31), which in turn informs the relationship between *naturalistic* theory (dominated by empirical research) and *normative* practice (governed by 'practical' knowledge), and perhaps more fundamentally between *fact* and *value*: what 'is' and what 'ought to be'.

Secondly, the appeal to bodies of knowledge as distinct and 'solid' – evidence-based, research-informed and cohesively integral – downplays the contestations at work within such bodies. 'Even in social work', Pavelová argues, 'the basic feature of pluralism becomes the existence of manifoldness and disparity, which often complement each other, but many times also exclude each other, or eventually at least contradict each other' (2014: 11). Noting the different 'ontological, epistemological and political assumptions' at work in the forms of social work (and in particular the differences between 'mainstream' and 'critical' social work), Cynthia Gallop notes that:

> the tension between these divergent understandings has also shaped the practice of social work. However, the growing neoliberal momentum toward theories and practices that bring order, predictability, and cohesion to our profession has begun to tip the balance in the social work profession in a manner that has had many in the field questioning *who we are*, and *what we actually do*. (Gallop 2013: 2, my emphasis)

Thus, while the EPAS state that social workers should understand 'scientific *and* ethical approaches to knowledge' (2008: 5, my emphasis), Gallop's political analysis seems to suggest that there is much to be debated regarding the nature of this 'and', which renders any simplistic or descriptive answer to her question about what social workers 'actually do' unsatisfactory. Framing social workers as *users* of theory, without articulating the way in which such theories presuppose particular senses of selfhood, seems only to perpetuate Taylor's problem of 'knowing where I stand'.

> **Thinking through Practice**
>
> In his work on social work values, Banks tracks the history of this ethical side of practitioners' capabilities. He argues that there 'is not one commonly agreed and coherent set of principles of social work', and while certain 'basic or first order' principles are identifiable – respect for self-determination, promotion of welfare or well-being, equality and distributive justice – 'none of these [...] is straightforward in meaning or implication for practice' (Banks 2000: 116–7). Furthermore, there can be conflicts between the content of the social worker's relationship with service users (the traditional focus of social work values), and the context of practice (such as 'social control' or 'resource-rationing') which carries its own set of ethical duties (119).
>
> Do you think that the ethical basis of social work is an example of Taylor's problem of 'knowing where I stand'? Are the 'ethical approaches' the EPAS refer to easier to outline than the 'scientific approaches'?

Training to be an 'I'

The plethora of accounts of what the self is, which continues to expand throughout modernity – simply think of the range of moral, psychosocial, therapeutic and consumer 'selves' that inhabit social work practice, often simultaneously – seems to problematise Gallop's question being answered in any straightforwardly descriptive way. When we ask the question of 'who am I?' or 'what is the nature of "the self" in social work practice?', we will inevitably look at the ever-widening range of theories that sit on the resource pile of the social work student, educator and/or practitioner. In doing so we are calling on another idea of the self: the self as a 'critical thinker', who applies balanced reasoning in order to question and challenge accepted forms of knowledge. Thus, the simple route through the tensions raised above is to appeal to a rational actor who is capable of choosing the appropriate self-resource – naturalistic or normative, material or spiritual, etc. – in the appropriate instance.

It is sometimes difficult to avoid the sense that laying out more and more theories for the discerning social worker to purvey is not unlike the displaying of all those different models of mobile phones or televisions across superstore shelves. This similarity is often overlooked, because there is an assumed dignity to 'critical thinking' that governs not just social work education, but education across the board. Increasingly, however, there is a risk of this assumption going unquestioned (see McBeath and Webb 2002). The ethicist and theologian Stanley Hauerwas summarised this disquieting idea with a short quip about the film *Dead Poets Society*. Hauerwas reminds us of how the lead character, played by Robin Williams, is commended for challenging the apparently unthinking authoritarianism of a private school, and encouraging students to overcome their resistance, to think for themselves and to realise their potential. But *why* is this commendable, Hauerwas asks?

The idea of individual autonomy is so ingrained in our sense of 'good practice', that it absorbs a whole range of ideas, ideals and ideologies which are not *necessarily* conducive to 'critical thinking'. Indeed, this example of 'radical' teaching makes for a good film because of its 'appeal to what anyone would think upon reflection' (Hauerwas 2010: 42). But while this appeal may be due to some innate shared understanding of the power of rational thinking, with a sharp about-turn Hauerwas suggests otherwise:

> I cannot think of a more conformist and suicidal message in modernity than that we should encourage students to make up their own minds. That is simply to ensure that they will be good conformist consumers in a capitalist economy by assuming now that ideas are but another product that you get to choose on the basis of your arbitrary likes and dislikes. To encourage students to think for themselves is therefore a sure way to avoid any meaningful disagreement. (Hauerwas 2010: 43)

Thinking through Practice

How do you understand Hauerwas's term 'meaningful disagreement' here? How do you discern meaningful disagreement from other forms of disagreement, and is this something that is of worth to social work practice?

In short, we need to be aware of the remarkable similarity between the 'critical thinker', who engages with theorists as an active interlocutor, and a 'critical consumer', who simply works through each theory until they find the one which satisfies them the best. Once the exercise of rationality substitutes purposive valuing with brute calculation, we are no longer 'thinking' but 'buying'. Once the assumption that an 'authentic individual' equates to an 'individual who chooses' takes such a hold of our thinking that it ceases to be questioned, then the significance of *what choice is made* is lost. But the moment of this loss is often concealed, due to the extent to which the 'prevailing ideology of Western capitalist societies' celebrates individualism and freedom as not only existential attributes of the self, but also core moral values (Banks 2000: 112). As Banks argues, this is reflected in the focus within social work values on the content of the social worker–service user relationship, rather than its context. But more than this: the freedom of Western modernity is itself ambiguous, in this sense, as it is both an act of *choice*, and a way to *truth*. This ambiguity is precisely how the idea of freedom eludes critique.[1]

While Hauerwas is writing from a different context, the point translates: the importance of teaching social workers 'critical thinking' is not *simply* so that they can 'think for themselves'. Thinking cannot be naively separated from the question of who we are; and who we are cannot be separated from the question of what we do, and why we do it. Hauerwas is critical of the idea that self-understanding can be treated *separately* from the contours of the self's development in and around its surroundings – whether these surroundings are material, social, or moral. The problem with *Dead Poets Society* is the 'critical thinking' that each student discovers is so familiar, it suggests a kind of universality: that deep down, we are all rational consumers.

But if critical thinking is to be of any value, it must be able to question this kind of familiarity. In this sense, the very language of identity is misleading, as it tends to presume an immediate and knowable 'self' which precedes the choices it makes. Our grammar, as Nietzsche once noted, requires we speak with an 'I', whether we know what that 'I' is or not. 'Thus', Hauerwas continues, '*training* is so important, because training involves the formation of the self [...] that will, if done well, provide people with virtues necessary to be able to make reasoned judgement' (43, my emphasis). Making a judgement, then – negotiating between the scientific and the ethical, the technical and the practical, the interventionist or the therapeutic, and so on – is not simply about making a 'choice'. It is not a fragmentary or arbitrary exercise, but instead involves seeing the self in terms of its development of virtues. At which point, we seem to come around in a circle: for how do we know which are the *right* virtues? Aren't we back to the problem of proficiencies again, where the social work student is required to follow possibly conflicting virtues? For Charles Taylor, this problem arises only because of the misguided path that the philosophy of identity – and its subsequent socio-cultural manifestations – has taken. Instead, he argues that we need to understand the self in terms of a concept that has been much-maligned in modern thinking: the concept of *authenticity*.

The malaises of identity

Authenticity is an ambiguous word, however. Taylor identifies two senses in which authenticity has been used in modern philosophy, both of which he sees as fundamentally flawed. First, there is a 'scientific' sense of authentic: which means, straightforwardly, the primacy of what is 'really there' as opposed to what is not. From this the naturalistic, disengaged ground, there is, in fact, no need for distinguishing between 'authentic' and 'inauthentic' if the correct methods and procedures are followed for discerning what the world is like, and describing it accurately. The self of the natural sciences is 'disengaged' in this sense: it is, effectively, an object amongst others. Second, there is a 'romantic' sense of authenticity, which is diametrically opposed to the scientific view: it is the idea that authenticity rests in 'being true to myself and my own particular way of being' (Taylor 1994: 28). Against the idea of a deterministic world whose workings can be revealed through repeated experiment, the romanticist sense of authenticity is located in our indeterminate freedom to act, create and express as we please (Taylor 1989: 495). While opposed in kind, the two sit on the same continuum: on the one end, an objective, outward sense of 'how things are' (the naturalist view), and on the other, a subjective, inward sense of freedom (the romanticist view). It is such a self that demands a kind of self-determining freedom which resists external impositions and allows one to 'decide for oneself' without influence (Taylor 1991: 27). And if the natural sciences provide us with no moral framework – in other words, if David Hume (1985) was correct that it is a fallacy to derive an 'ought' from an 'is' – then it is this self-determining sense of authenticity which provides us with the 'ethical' or 'artistic' side of the social work self.

While both may provide goals of self-fulfilment – clear and accurate knowledge for the naturalistic view; free self-expression for the romanticist – they both do this without any sense of the *relational* demands of others, or without any sense of aspiration beyond the human 'individual'; and as such, both are ultimately self-defeating, as these two conditions are fundamental to realising authenticity (Taylor 1991: 35). Taylor describes this self-defeat in terms of three key 'malaises' that have accompanied the development of modernity: individualism, instrumental reason, and soft despotism. Each captures a particular sense of loss: individualism leads to the loss of meaning and moral horizons; the use of instrumental reason requires the loss of end goals as a focus for action; and the resignation to soft despotism signifies a loss of freedom (1991: 10). At the same time, we can see from considering each in the context of social work that these losses arise from what would otherwise appear to be advances in society:

1. *Individualism.* The emergence of an individual as a rational agent, separable from their social and spiritual contexts, was one of the most fundamental and significant outcomes of the age of Enlightenment. Industrialisation grew not only from the rights of the wealthy individual to pursue profit, but also the lower classes to sell their own labour in order to accrue wages. The machines and assembly lines of the factory removed agrarian societies from their dependence on the land; as did the canals, railways and roads. In this sense, the triumph of individualism is the central motif of the modern age.

    Of course, the rise of individualism is often the target of critique by radical and critical social work. If individualism promoted freedom, correspondingly the individualisation of social problems – poverty, poor education, ill health – legitimised blaming the marginalised and disadvantaged members of society for their own problems. While early social work initiatives such as the Charity Organisation Society in the UK were explicitly focused on the problems of the individual (see Pierson 2011: 33), individualisation continued to be a source of tension throughout the twentieth century: for example, Specht and Courtney (1994) criticise the development of social work in the US for its privileging clinical 'scientific' stature of individualist practice as the *de facto* model of knowledge. The individualisation of the task of social work echoes Taylor's claim that 'the dark side of individualism is a centring on the self, which both flattens and narrows our lives, makes them poorer in meaning, and less concerned with others or society' (1991: 4).

2. *Instrumental Reason.* The malaise of individualism, and its concern with the loss of meaning, links to that of instrumental reason, which identifies a loss in our methods of thinking itself. It is 'the kind of rationality we draw on when we calculate the most economical application of means to a given end. Maximum efficiency,

the best cost-output ration, is its measure of success' (Taylor 1991: 5). Such a concern about the role of 'instrumental reason' has been raised by Marxist and radical social workers since as far back as the 1960s, criticising the emphasis on individual caseload, a reliance on managerialist strategies to service user problems, and a resigned acceptance of the power structures that social work operates within: it has 'grown along with a disengaged model of the human subject' characterised in the way that economic rationality has become 'one of the most prestigious forms of reason in our culture' (1991: 101–2). But Taylor wants to go a little further here, by unpacking how the reliance on instrumental reason can develop from what, initially at least, may seem like an act of liberation.

> [T]he order of things [...] can be redesigned with their consequences for the happiness and well-being of individuals as our goal. The yardstick that henceforth applies is that of instrumental reason. Similarly, once the creatures that surround us lose the significance that accrued to their place in the chain of being, they are open to being treated as raw materials or instruments for our projects. (Taylor 1991: 5)

This is not simply an echo of Marx and Engels' prophecy of 1848 that, with rapid industrial expansion, 'all that is solid will melt into air'. For these questions are frequently met with a plurality of both 'scientific' and 'ethical' theories which *might* answer such a question: to the extent that, as Pavelová observes, 'it is impossible to find or build one all-embracing theory which could explain everything and find answers to all questions, including prognoses of socially undesirable phenomena and problems in a society'. In this sense, 'Lyotard's so-called collapse of the "Grand Narrative" has fully affected social work as well' (Pavelová 2014: 11). The neoliberal momentum which we have seen both Hauerwas and Gallop allude to is not simply towards an ordered and predictable world per se, but also an ordered range of theories that, *by virtue* of that ordering, all become much of a muchness in terms of value and propriety. When the search for identity rests upon a free market of available accounts of the self, the question of *how to choose* is often left assumed, or unnoticed.

3. *Soft Despotism.* Of course, if we cease to look for what matters within our use of reasoning, and assume instead that we are acting out heuristic devices and decision-making processes, then we run the risk of, at best, allowing what matters to be dictated by something other than our own sense of worth; at worst, we succumb to the sense that there are no more battles worth fighting any more, as we lack a coherent sense of why one approach or model is better or worse than another, beyond procedural requirements. This is not to say, it should be noted, that we don't use heuristic devices and decision-making processes – these are vital, and inevitable, tools of practice. But when we downplay the *evaluative* role built within reasoning, we effectively sign over the value of what we do to someone or something else. Perhaps nowhere is this contestation more heated than the progression of the personalisation agenda in the UK: John

Burton, for example, argues forcefully that the individualisation of the vulnerable under the mantra of 'personalisation' is an oxymoron: '"Personalisation" is a bureaucratic word for a bureaucratic response to the political failure of social care' (2010: 301). Yet, the language of personalisation – the rights of the individual, and the accompanying reformulation of service-based relationships as financial transactions (Barnes 2006: 147) – can serve to obscure what Banks terms a 'new authoritarianism': the language of consumerism masks the power differentials that remain within welfare provision, and 'calling the user a consumer also serves to hide the fact of social worker as controller' (2000: 116).

Thinking through Practice

Taylor suggests that these malaises of individualism, instrumental reason and soft despotism are well known to us, and this familiarity can lead to us ignoring their significance. How do these emerge within the context of social work education? Is Taylor right to think that their familiarity is a risk worth attending to?

Knowing how to choose: naturalistic identity vs narrative identity

These malaises, Taylor argues, result in a social and philosophical account of the self which is deeply *proceduralist*. The paradox they result in, however, is that they reflect ideals of human autonomy, based upon the rationalisation of human nature, yet *also* suffer from a normative indeterminacy (Taylor 1994: 38). With no discernible 'order' of things to draw upon, our only source for distinguishing between values and norms beyond 'following the forms' is precisely our own *contingency* – that is, our sense of being an individual. But this means, somewhat uncomfortably, that the source of our values – spuriously described as our 'freedom to choose' – is simply the social, cultural and historical determinants that distinguish us from anybody else.

Taylor suggests that there may yet be a model of an 'authentic self' which challenges the social determinist models which see the self as produced from the social, economic, scientific and bureaucratic structures around it; as well as the flattening mantras of postmodernism, or relativist individualism based on the arbitrary pursuit of 'free choice'. The original goal of postulating an 'authentic self' is not *itself* misguided; indeed, it remains, for Taylor, the best way to overcome these malaises (1991: 56). We can explore his argument in terms of a clear opposition between the way the self is thought about: on the one hand, the proceduralist sense of self is fundamentally embodied in what we will term a 'post-Lockean' account of who we are; and against this, the likes of Taylor put forward a 'narrative' account of self.[2] By briefly recounting the post-Lockean 'third person' view of the self, we can articulate Taylor's own 'first person' account, before turning again to the question of the self-in-training in a social work context.

Post-Lockean accounts begin from the starting points laid out by the seventeenth century philosopher John Locke. For Locke, self-identity was based on psychological continuity. We judge the identity of material objects (chairs, tables etc.) by the fact that they have the same material substance. While the way in which their materials are arranged may change over time, so long as it remains the same materials, it remains the same object. For living things, however, this doesn't work, as the material substance of, say, a human being is changing all the time. If we look at an adult, and ask if they are the same person as they were when they were a child, we cannot simply compare their skin, hair and organs, as these will all be different. So in this sense, to identify ourselves involves looking beyond the merely physical (e.g. our bodies) to the sense of what organises and unifies all the different parts of a living thing (Locke 1993: 174–7). We can, of course, speak of 'humans' *just* in terms of their physical or biological continuity, as we do when we refer to humanity as, say, a species. But for Locke, while biological continuity describes a 'human', self-identity involves speaking of 'persons'. It is a forensic term, relevant to legal disputes, or questions of moral worthiness. For persons, the organising principle is *consciousness*:

> *Self* is that conscious thinking thing (whatever substance made up of, whether spiritual or material, simple or compounded, it matters not) which is sensible or conscious of pleasure and pain, capable of happiness or misery, and so is concerned for *itself*, as far as that consciousness extends. (Locke 1993: 186)

Hence, psychological continuity – consciousness and memory – is what makes us 'us'.[3] On this account, it is perfectly possible for someone to be the same man over a course of 20 years, but not the same person.[4] Indeed (Locke argues) if we cut a finger off, we would not imagine that the finger would become 'us' and the rest of our body would cease to be 'us'. Note, as well, that Locke is deliberately vague as to what this 'substance' is – he is not, like Descartes, a dualist who believes that the mind and body are separate things. His account remains fundamentally empirical, as it is based on the evidence of our senses: he is referring to selfhood as a certain 'sensation' of which we are all aware.

If this seems slightly abstract, then this is precisely the point: for Locke, and those who have followed his line of thought (see, for example, Parfit 1984; see also Martin and Barresi 2003), the important point is to isolate the fundamental sense of what the 'self' is, and that can be applied to any situation; and more to the point, in a situation-by-situation manner. It is a waymark that aims to cut through the complexity of the contexts we otherwise find ourselves in, and allows us to differentiate and disengage the identical aspects of our existence (who we are) from the evaluative ones (what we do). So, to return to our initial problem of the self in tension within social work education, the question would be how do we identify a sense of self amid contradictory or conflicting demands as to what this self should be? How do we maintain a sense of identity when the act of training itself involves questioning core values, improving skills, and adding competencies? And the answer, for the post-Lockean[5] view, is that the self is a series of related, continuous states of consciousness, that link together effectively through the memory of past states. So long as there is psychological continuity, there is a self.

The significance of this view is that it speaks to an ideal of *disengaged reason*; a view which becomes increasingly persuasive within a fragmented and atomistic account of the world around us. Hence, we saw before the emphasis on 'critical thinking' as a disengaged activity: within social work education, this involved the lining up of an array of possible theories and bodies of evidence in order to decide on which 'fitted' the circumstances. The only tangible concern of the self-in-training *vis-à-vis* self-identity is its self-possession: that there is a thing that we know is 'us' now, and that we still have in the next 'now', and the next. It is this which allows the self to transcend the different theoretical and practical contexts to emerge as an informed and knowledgeable social work practitioner. Taylor links this approach specifically to a number of corresponding ideas surrounding identity, knowledge and values:

> The ideal of disengagement defines a certain – typically modern – notion of freedom, as the ability to act on one's own, without outside interference or subordination to outside authority. It defines its own peculiar notion of human dignity, closely connected to freedom. And these in turn are linked to ideals of efficacy, power, unperturbability, which for all their links with earlier ideals are original with modern culture.
>
> The great attraction of these ideals, all the more powerful in that this understanding of the agent is woven into a host of modern practices – economic, scientific, technological, psycho-therapeutic, and so on – lends great weight and credence to the disengaged image of the self. (Taylor 1985: 5)

Thinking through Practice

Parton and O'Byrne assert that 'by definition we as individuals are never "disinterested" and cannot escape our involvement in life and our attempts to understand and make it meaningful' (2000: 176).

To what extent does social workers' lack of 'disinterest' lead them away from a 'disengaged' sense of self? What are the benefits to being an interested practitioner, while maintaining a disengaged concept of self? What are the problems?

The problem is not the methods of the natural sciences themselves, but their 'illusionary pretensions to define the totality of our lives as agents' (1985: 7). Applying such methods to the domain of the self produces an 'atomistic' sense of identity (and the knowledge, freedom and values which are embedded within it), which casts the individual as 'metaphysically independent of society' (8). The fragmentation and atomisation of the social field which fuels the malaises of modernity is facilitated on two, interrelated fronts. Not only does it stem from the socio-cultural abandonment of any unifying narratives of what counts as 'good', 'right' or 'valued' – in this sense, Taylor re-states the communitarian arguments we saw in Chapter 2 – but also from the insistence on a particular form of epistemology governing what we know about social practice: 'the more we are led to interpret ourselves in the light of the disengaged picture, to define our identity by this, the more the connected epistemology of naturalism will seem right and proper to us' (6). Indeed, Andrew Sayer has agreed that the social sciences in general have struggled with acknowledging that 'people's relation to the world is one of concern' (Sayer 2011: 1): whether this is due to methodological assumptions that people act in 'terms of self-interest, or norm-following, or habitual action, or discursive constitution' (8), or due to wariness of the language of ethics (what we *ought* to do) conflicting with the language of empirical inquiry (what *is* happening). However, for Sayer, the 'distinction between *is* and *ought*, that has dominated thinking about values in social science, allows us to overlook the missing middle, the centrality of *evaluation*' (4, my emphasis).

It is this missing middle that the narrative view of identity picks up.[6] For Taylor, evaluation will necessarily involve a form of authenticity – a sense of value that transcends specific contexts – to guide it. Patrick Stokes summarises the position of narrative identity as this:

> the self exists (whether as a real object or fictional construct) as a temporally-extended form of narrative-qualified continuity between psychological and physical events. However, instead of merely determining the conditions under which a self can be said to persist between two different points in time, as most post-Lockean identity theorists do, narrative theorists generally add the qualification that 'we need to think of ourselves as temporally extended *wholes*.' Narratives have an overall shape and trajectory, which gives them a unity that goes beyond mere continuity between discrete points in time. (Stokes 2008: 657)

The self is thus always evaluating itself in terms of its narrative continuity: humans 'are not neutral, punctual objects; they exist only in a certain space of questions […] [which] touch on the nature of the good that I orient myself by and on the way I am placed in relation to it' (Taylor 1989: 50). Self-identity is thus formed by forming narrative links between what matters to us. And what matters is not a subjective or arbitrary choice, as 'one cannot be a self on one's own' (36): the self only ever exists in relation to others (whether such relations are happy or unhappy, familial or distant, and so on), and so what matters to it is embedded within these 'webs of interlocution': who is speaking to it and who it speaks back to (and, as Sayer reminds us, we must be careful not to over-emphasise *speech* alone, and remember that 'our identity is also shaped by being held, loved, hurt, ignored, shamed, played with, celebrated, etc.' (2011: 120)).

Such relations present themselves not as discrete moments or given points in time, but rather as 'constitutive concerns' that shape both our awareness of 'who we are' as a self, and the evaluations that self makes (Taylor 1989: 49). While the post-Lockean account 'simply recounts events between two given points of time'; the narrative account depends on a beginning and an end for its essential shape. As Stokes continues, 'if we want to see our actions to be intelligible to ourselves, on this line, then we must see them as embedded in some larger narrative, which in turn will make sense with reference to yet larger narratives' (Stokes 2008: 658), and so on until we have what Stokes calls the 'whole life intelligibility thesis'. By understanding our identity as an act of self-interpretation, we form a teleological unity that makes sense of who we are and what we should do. This allows for a sense of authenticity which the 'third person' perspective does not: the psychological continuity theorist looks at two separate times which require re-identification ('what licenses us in saying self A at one o'clock is the same self as self B at two o'clock?'), while the narrative perspective asks a fundamentally hermeneutic question: 'under what description can I characterise this past or future person as being an appropriate object of my self-regarding concern?' This, then, provides a qualitative link between 'who I am' and 'what I do' within social work practice that Gallop raised earlier. As Anthony Rudd argues, to 'understand any action is to situate it in a context which renders it intelligible, and that context is itself rendered intelligible by the wider narrative of the agent's life to which it contributes' (2001: 138). For the narrative theory of the self, *every* attempt to think through the self does this necessarily, even the post-Lockean. But approaches which emphasise the self as disengaged are using a half-formed or inconsistent account of what this wider narrative is; because understanding the self is, for Taylor, fundamentally about negotiating other people, perspectives, and attitudes, as well as what they mean to us.

The narrative account of identity thus seems to provide a way through the apparent contradictions in the idea of the self-in-training within social work education. Rather than looking for a procedurally reductive starting point, it suggests that identity is formed through the gradual emergence of a horizon of authenticity, which ontologically precedes the distinction between 'science' and 'ethics' that the proficiencies describe (much in the way that, as we saw in Chapter 1, Gadamer's interpretative horizon preceded any specific, concrete interpretation). Within this horizon, the assumptions of selfhood at work in both can be fully articulated and measured; and their 'usefulness' is not the result of impartial 'critical thinking' – whereby rational deliberation is seen as a disengaged, procedural instrument – but rather the best expression of this authenticity. In short: when we reflect on our decision-making and activities across time (and across training), it reveals not simply what 'works', but more fundamentally what *matters*.[7] Webb thus comments that, in a social work context, Taylor's position:

> not only reinstates the value of ideas and conceptually-based professional opinion, but places them at the head of any pyramid of understanding for reaching decisions in social work. Thus it is the social workers conception of how things are, rather than the evidential facts *per se* which determine actions.
> (Webb 2001: 66)

Against authenticity? Some problems for Taylor

I said at the start of the chapter that the particular perspective of the self-in-training raises some specific problems for this view, though. I want to raise three here.

1. Firstly, given that we are unlikely to hold a 'whole life intelligibility thesis' from the off, and particularly not in the field of training, what is to stop this account of who we are lapsing into some kind of relativism based on a student social worker's 'instincts' or 'common sense'? How does it not return us to the sense of authenticity based on 'what I feel deep down inside me' which we were trying to avoid? In short, what *accountability* does narrative identity have?[8] The post-Lockean tradition, not to mention much work in the philosophy of mind and cognitive science, argued that the self could be examined using the same tools as that of the natural sciences, and as such had a clear 'method' to rely on. But narrative identity does not seem to offer this clarity.
2. Secondly, Taylor could be criticised for over-intellectualising the basic lived conditions of being an 'I': he exaggerates the importance of morality in the constitution of our selves (Flanagan 1993). As a result, his account of authenticity seems to over-emphasise personal development over and above structural axes of subordination (see Fraser 2003). The freedom that Taylor argues for is denied to some, and not to others, and without a clear analysis of the *institutional* forms of power at work in the shaping of the self, it remains naively optimistic. From a social work perspective, Garrett argues that subscribing too quickly to *either* Taylor or Fraser's political philosophies 'risks mistakenly casting social work as existing *outside* of the dominant social and economic relations that characterise the times in which we live' (2013: 177). Instead, social work students need to recognise how their identity is already articulated by extra-moral concerns: for example, the acute financial demands on not only practice placement organisations, but also on training institutions, which place specific boundaries on the narratives a student might form. More broadly, how, on a practical level, might a social work student 'narrate' the fact that social work's state funding will often render the social worker complicit in many of the instrumental procedures that Taylor critiques (see Garrett 2013: 170)? What defence, for that matter, does narrative identity provide against the longstanding problem that celebrating an occupation for its 'moral calling' can easily serve as an underhanded excuse for increased workload and less pay?
3. Thirdly, the idea of the narrative self is problematic because it simply multiplies the problem of identity rather than solves it: the self as *narrated* depends upon the self as *narrating*. Narrative identity seems to confuse where 'we' actually are. Furthermore, Vice (2003) notes that narrative accounts of the self tend to employ fairly *conservative* accounts of narrative as a form: narrative is invoked here for its sense of *unity*, rather than its broken plotlines, or ironic subversion: a narrative self is not based on *Memento* or *The Usual Suspects*. The self within

social work education provides a richer context for discerning a clear arch-narrative: for this self-interpreting, evaluative self is also aware of *being* evaluated, both by educators and service users within field education, and always within a context of historical tensions over what 'matters' within the profession, which in turn guides its proficiencies.

All of these criticisms, in different ways, circle around the question of evaluation – how we evaluate our own 'narrative' as being appropriate to the training we are undertaking or the profession we belong to, how we evaluate the practicality of that narrative, and how we evaluate the concept of narrative as complex and misshapen rather than risking platitudinous celebrations of some kind of 'life journey'. So we need to say a little more about the nature of evaluation within the narrative account, and see if this helps to respond to these objections.

The problem with objection 1 is that it leaves a distinction between 'fact' and 'value' intact which is upheld by the post-Lockean view, but not the narrative view. It is confusing the sense of 'good' as Taylor employs it with the definitions of 'values' that are embedded within the naturalistic approach to self: whether this is a view of values as something that floats above the world of factual science, or the 'romanticist' version of authenticity which is defined only by opposing the objectivity of naturalism with an equally disengaged subjectivism. But Taylor is specifically arguing against a relativistic or therapeutic sense of 'authenticity'. He is a moral realist: he believes that narratives constructed to suit the individual will not aim towards 'goods' that are as 'good' as those that are shared and agreed across the relations between the individual self and other selves and perspectives. The difference, then, is less one of 'fact' and 'value', and more one of 'weak' and 'strong' evaluation.

Thinking through Practice

It is often the case that learning what Parton and O'Byrne referred to as the 'psy' disciplines is disagreeable to some students, who would rather focus on the practical, hands-on business than learning theories of, say, social psychology. What reasons might they have for deciding this?

- It may be that they simply find the prospect of learning such theories daunting: they tend to challenge our common sense judgements on the world (see Taylor 1985: 92), and making the world strange is not the most comfortable of activities.
- It may be that their field experience has returned a negative view of such 'theorising' and its use in the particular organisations they have worked in. Their supervisor may stress that 'getting the job done' is more important than theorising it. Thus, the rejection of any 'science' of practice is part of their socialisation into the social work environment.

> - It may be that they find the methodological assumptions at work in the studies which support this knowledge questionable: the use of experimental conditions, for example, or the use of a particular demographic of participant that does not coincide neatly with that of their service user group. Based on the values that their education has instilled in them to this point, they see the benefits of it as a resource, but not as the final word on their practice.
>
> Of these reasons, which do you think is a 'weak' evaluation, and which is a 'strong' one? What are the differences?

For Taylor, evaluation based on what we happen to feel like at the time – such as the first reason – constitutes a 'weak evaluation': it makes no larger claim other than seeming to be right in that particular instant. This may well involve utilising available facts – the student may opt for the most basic introduction to psychology, for example, in order to make a reasoned effort at 'just doing enough' – but the evaluation of what the right thing to do is made within and for the purpose of the present moment.

Making a decision in terms of its *worth*, however, constitutes a 'strong evaluation'. This is what seems to be going on in the second and third reasons. In these, the student is attempting to measure and order the effect and impact of the theory on their working practice. However, they arrive at different conclusions. The second seems to echo aspects of objection 2 above: that structural conditions regulate the extent to which we self-interpret. The reasons could be manifold, of course: the student's own background may mean that they are unfamiliar with the style and prose of academic psychology, for example.

What is the difference between the second and third reasons, then? For Taylor, the difference rests on the measure being used to assess what is of worth. While there are 'goods' apparent in both the importance of socialisation into a working environment, and the understanding of the broader context within which social work knowledge is formed, strong evaluations deal with the overarching 'good' that we use to relate these smaller goods into a coherent narrative surrounding our identity. He uses the term 'hypergood' for 'goods which are not only incomparably more important than others but provide the standpoint from which these must be weighed, judged, decided about' (1989: 63). In other words, these lay the foundation for the intelligibility of our narrative. Taylor's own primary example is 'a notion of universal justice and/or benevolence, in which all human beings are treated equally with respect. Regardless of race, class, sex, culture, religion' (64).

Importantly, a hypergood is not only more important than other goods (the pursuit of wealth or happiness, for example), but also actively critical of them. We find these hypergoods by looking for the 'best available', which entails the kind of 'meaningful disagreement' that Hauerwas mentioned earlier. Ultimately, the strength of the second and third reasons for the social work student's aversion to psychology is decided by the extent to which it withstands challenges to the sense they make; or, in Taylor's words:

> Our conviction that we have grown morally can be challenged by another. It may, after all, be illusion. And then we argue; and arguing here is contesting between interpretations of what I have been living. (Taylor 1989: 72)

Hypergoods are a source of conflict, and not necessarily comfort: the fact that they precede any 'facts' necessitates this. For example, while Taylor argues that his notion of universal justice is widely adhered to in our civilisation, it arises by actively superseding 'earlier, less adequate views' (64). The importance of hypergoods is, then, that they denounce other, less worthy, moral sentiments or cultural 'goods'. As such, they carry with them the transcendence that the disengaged self promised, while remaining situated within our social practices. Our sense of hypergood 'engenders a pitiless criticism' of any values we have which do not live up to its standards (69). Hence, his concern with 'soft despotism' is precisely the obscuring of what is 'good' about the goods we follow: in the case of the personalisation agenda, for example, where Banks (2000) earlier critiqued the language of rights as obscuring the lack of universal respect; in the case of our social work student's aversion to psychology, the task is to measure their interpretation against the strongest 'good' available, and to use this to discern whether their reasoning is overly-pragmatic, overly-intellectual, or otherwise.

To this extent, I do not see objection 2 above as a fatal one. Of course, Taylor veers towards a moralistic, intellectualist stance on identity, because that is the web of interlocution he works within. In works such as *The Sources of the Self*, Taylor is articulating what matters to the self from the perspective of the history of philosophy. From the perspective of social work education, there may well be much more articulation of particular structural and ideological determinants that shape what 'matters' in that context. The question becomes: from what perspective can such determinants be articulated *except* through the self as situated, engaged and narrated? Whereas, for the naturalist position, this would be done from absolute, fixed or disengaged positions, for Taylor 'there cannot be such considerations. My perspective is defined by the moral intuitions I have, by what I am morally moved by. If I abstract from this, I become incapable of understanding any moral argument at all' (1989: 73). It is in this way that social theory breaks from the methods of the natural sciences, Taylor argues, because (echoing Gadamer) there is 'always a *pre-theoretical* understanding of what is going on among the members of a society, which is formulated in the descriptions of the self and other which are involved in the institutions and practices of that society' (1985: 93, my emphasis). It is because our relations with others, and therefore our pre-theoretical understanding, are real – in other words, they have their own effective-historical dimension, as they are born from our concrete relations with others – that it is possible to reason and argue about them. Thus we could respond to the criticism that the focus on the 'first person' sense of self omits the structural realities of social work practice by suggesting that a corollary of discussing 'hypergoods' is to also discuss what prevents their achievement (see László

2008). Likewise, articulating fully the nature of these determinant structures of self – the relationship between their history, power and significance – *from* a 'first person' perspective allows us to evaluate how they are incorporated into our narrative selves. As Sayer remarks, 'strange though it may seem to social science-trained ears, *this* is where we live – between the actual and the possible, between present flourishing and suffering and future possible flourishing or suffering' (2011: 18, my emphasis).

This point may go some way to answering objection 3 as well; the use of narrative as an account of the self is to emphasise that these narratives can be shared and agreed on, rather than to indulge in literary appropriation. Hence, the theory uses basic and universal features of story-telling: features that 'count as narratives in just about any context' (Currie 2010: 35). It is this core sense of narrative – in Goldie's words, 'a representation of events which is shaped, organized, and coloured, presenting those events, and the people involved in them, from a certain perspective or perspectives' (2012: 8) – which, Taylor argues, allows us to comprehend ourselves as inherently committed to and constituted by the concerns of others without dissolving, in the manner of postmodern critiques of identity, into a free-floating 'signifier'. There does, however, remain a sense in which this depends upon some assumptions that we have not yet made clear: for example, how such basic and universal narratives, however basic and universal, come to be known as such; and, conversely, the extent to which narrative organisation could be otherwise in terms of self-identity. There are perhaps echoes here of Habermas's critique of Gadamer's hermeneutics, which we explored in Chapter 1, for ignoring the prevalence of ideology in shaping what appears before us. But it is perhaps worth noting that Taylor would not be alone in drawing on such assumptions: they reflect the basic form of 'storying' that Larson and Sjöblom (2010) identify as core to the use of narrative methods across social work research, and that Philips *et al.* (2012) argue forms a core bridge between social work education and social work research: the communal act of 'telling stories' is a key part of the self-in-training.

Despite the challenges, at the heart of this debate over the philosophy of self is the case for a broader language to describe 'thinking', in order to reveal the conditions of terms such as 'critical', 'reflective', 'anti-oppressive' and so on. Otherwise, these terms remain surface gestures rather than part of a higher-order analysis, and the complexity of the social world is such that surface gestures rarely operate for long without encountering contradiction, tension or mutation. There are clear risks in using a simplistic vocabulary that glides deceptively over what is, within the multifaceted, polyphonic and plural world in which late modern social work inhabits, an often-contradictory notion. Taylor's challenge, in sum, is to re-engage with these surface phenomena: not to continue avoiding the risks of the grand metanarrative or sanctimonious clichés such as 'authenticity', but instead to articulate them in ways that are practically meaningful. Thus, whereas Clegg (1993) once warned against grand narratives within social theory, and called for greater attention to be given to local narratives of daily lives, for Taylor the direction of the narratives which shape our self is *necessarily* organised by a grand narrative – the task is to articulate it well.

Thinking through Practice

We noted earlier that Stephen Webb cited Taylor as part of his critique of the application of evidence-based practice (EBP) within social work: where, for example, he asserts that 'if we want to understand why clients, or indeed, social workers, act as they do, we need to understand their conceptual thinking and not empirical evidence of controlled behaviours' (2001: 66). In a recent article on social work in the United States, Okpych and Yu have argued that EBP constitutes an 'empirically grounded practice paradigm' (2014: 39) formed from the contextual and political demands made on practice, which moves social work away from paradigms that were previously morality-based (such as the early charity-based work of the 1860s to the early 1900s) and authority-based (the development of the 'profession' of social work from 1915 to the 1960s).

While acknowledging that evidence-based practice is not 'the only option' to deal with the current demands for 'measurable accountability' within social work, they also suggest that:

> philosophical skepticism, practical barriers, and practitioner ambivalence appear as barriers [...] to empirically grounded practice. [...] At this point in time, it is hard to discern whether these barriers and forms of resistance are more accurately viewed as surmountable obstacles to be overcome or as indications that EBP in its current forms is an inadequate or unrealistic paradigmatic response to the crisis of increased accountability. (Okpych and Yu 2014: 40)

How convincing do you find Taylor's argument regarding strong evaluation in respect of Okpych and Yu's observation here?

How might the objections we raised at the start of this section respond in turn to the defence of Taylor's case outlined above, that the self within social work education should be considered as a moral, rather than scientific, entity?

Notes

1. It is also, in many senses, a route to understanding how the 'neoliberal momentum' which Gallop earlier referred to offers 'cohesion and order' which is, almost paradoxically, unworkable in a social work context.
2. This sense of a 'narrative self' is not, it should be noted, the same thing as the use of narrative as a therapeutic form in practice (see, for example, Freeman 2011); although practical application and philosophical framework can, and frequently do, interlink.
3. For an interesting discussion on how the psychological and biological accounts of persons and humans differ in terms of the applied case of working with dementia, see DeGrazia (1999).
4. This view has a number of separate implications, all of interest – for example, it suggests that if we can't remember being 'us' at a previous point then we are not technically the same

'person'. So if we committed a crime, but then suffered a bout of irreversible amnesia, it would be senseless to punish us. It also allows for two different 'people' to occupy the same body.
5   The difference between the Lockean and post-Lockean view is based on modifications to Locke's initial arguments in their entirety, which we do not need to attend to in this context. Post-Lockean views maintain the basic structure of Locke's thinking on the self as being based on psychological continuity, which is all that is relevant to our discussion here.
6   It should be noted that while Taylor's views on the self are similar throughout his career, he does not always use the language of 'narrative identity' in the way we do here. For a more detailed survey of narrative themes within philosophical views on identity, see Atkins and MacKenzie (2010).
7   This, incidentally, is precisely why Taylor is critical of theories which may *appear* to resist the second 'malaise' of modernity – the primacy of instrumental reason – and in particular, the Critical Theory school of Marxist social thought, and Weber's notion of the 'iron cage' of coercive bureaucracy (Taylor 1989: 500), as these theories often fail to challenge the fundamental notion of *rationality* itself. Reasoning, for Taylor, is not simply a functional mechanism, but also evaluative.
8   There is a corollary reactionary argument to be made here regarding the role of science within social work practice itself, which was perhaps made most vociferously by Brian Sheldon (2001) in response to Webb's Taylor-inspired critique of evidence-based practice. But this objection is a weak one: it inserts a false dichotomy between 'fact' and 'value' – which we will discuss later – that wilfully ignores the point that Taylor is not critiquing 'science' itself. Rather, he is critiquing the hermeneutical starting point of naturalist philosophy, which leads to 'a bad philosophy of science' and, in turn, an uncertain science of the self.

References

Atkins, K. and MacKenzie, C. (eds.) (2010). *Practical Identity and Narrative Agency*. London: Routledge.
Banks, S. (2000). 'Social Work Values.' In Davies, C., Finlay, L. and Bullman, A. (eds), *Changing Practice in Health and Social Care*. London: Sage, pp. 112–20.
Barnes, M. (2006). *Caring and Social Justice*. Basingstoke: Palgrave Macmillan.
Basham, R.E. and Buchanan, F. R. (2009). 'A Survey Comparison of Career Motivations of Social Work and Business Students.' *Journal of Social Work Education*, 45, 2, 187–208.
Brewer, C. and Lait, J. (1980). *Can Social Work Survive?* London: Maurice Temple Smith.
Burton, J. (2010). 'Call it Personalisation if you Like': The Realities and Dilemmas of Organising Care in a Small Rural Community.' *Journal of Social Work Practice*, 24, 3, 301–13.
Camilleri, P. (1999). 'Social Work and its Search for Meaning: Theories, Narratives and Practice.' In Pease, B. and Fook, J. (eds), *Transforming Social Work Practice*. London: Routledge, pp. 25–39.
Clegg, S. (1993). 'Narrative Power and Social Theory.' In Mumby, D. (ed.), *Narrative and Social Control*. London: Sage.
College of Social Work (2012). *Professional Capabilities Framework*. Available at http://www.tcsw.org.uk/pcf.aspx
Council of Social Work Education (2008). *Educational Policy and Accreditation Standards*. Available at http://www.cswe.org/File.aspx?id=41861
Currie, G. (2010). *Narratives and Narrators*. Oxford: Oxford University Press.
Daniel, C. and Quirros, L. (2010). 'Disrupting the Dominant Discourse: Rethinking Identity Development in Social Work Education and Practice.' *The International Journal of Diversity in Organisations, Communities and Nations*, 10, 4, 283–94.

DeGrazia, D. (1999). 'Advance Directives, Dementia, and "the Someone Else Problem",' *Bioethics*, 13, 373–91.
Descartes, R. (1986 [1641]). *Meditations on First Philosophy*. J. Cottingham (trans.). Cambridge: Cambridge University Press.
Dulmus, C. N. and Sowers, K. M. (2012). *The Profession of Social Work: Guided by History, Led by Evidence*. Oxford: Wiley Blackwell.
Earls Larrison, T. and Korr, W. (2013). 'Does Social Work Have a Signature Pedagogy?' *Journal of Social Work Education*, 49, 2, 194–206.
Edwards, P. (2002). 'Spiritual Themes in Social Work Counselling: Facilitating the Search for Meaning.' *Australian Social Work*, 5, 1, 78–87.
Flanagan, O. (1993). 'Identity and Strong and Weak Evaluation.' In Flanagan, O. and Rorty, A. (eds.), *Identity, Character and Morality*. Boston.MA: MIT Press, pp. 37–66.
Foucault, M. (1984). 'Truth and Power.' In Rabinow, P. (ed.), *The Foucault Reader*. London: Penguin, pp. 51–75.
Fraser, N. (2003). 'Social Justice in an Age of Identity Politics: Redistribution, Recognition and Participation.' In Fraser, N. and Honneth, A. (eds), *Redistribution or Recognition?* London: Verso, pp. 7–109.
Freeman, E. (2011). *Narrative Approaches in Social Work Practice: A Life Span, Culturally Centered, Strengths Perspective*. Springfield, IL: Charles C. Thomas.
Gallop, C. (2013). 'Knowing Nothing: Understanding New Critical Social Work Practice.' *Journal of Applied Hermeneutics*. Available at: http://jah.journalhosting.ucalgary.ca/jah/index.php/jah/article/view/44
Goldie, P. (2012). *The Mess Inside: Narrative, Emotion and the Mind*. Oxford: Oxford University Press.
Greene, R. (2008). 'Human Behaviour Theory, Person-in-Environment and Social Work Method.' In Green, R. (ed.), *Human Behaviour Theory and Social Work Practice*. New Brunswick, NJ: Transaction Publishers, pp. 1–24.
Hauerwas, S. (2010). 'How We Lay Bricks and Make Disciples.' In Bretherton, L. and Rook, R. (eds), *Living Out Loud*. Milton Keynes: Paternoster, pp. 39–59.
Hume, D. (1985 [1738]). *A Treatise of Human Nature*. London: Penguin.
Jennissen, T. and Lundy, C. (2011). *One Hundred Years of Social Work: A History of the Profession in English Canada, 1900–2000*. Waterloo, Ontario: Wilfrid Laurier University Press.
Larson, S. and Sjöblom, Y. (2010). 'Perspectives on Narrative Methods in Social Work Research.' *International Journal of Social Welfare*, 19, 272–80.
Lash, S. (1999). *Another Modernity, A Different Rationality*. Oxford: Blackwell.
László, J. (2008). *The Science of Stories: An Introduction to Narrative Psychology*. London: Routledge.
Locke, J. (1993 [1690]). *An Essay Concerning Human Understanding*. London: Everyman.
Lyotard, J-F. (1984). *The Postmodern Condition: A Report on Knowledge*. Manchester: Manchester University Press.
Marthinsen, E. and Skjefstad, N. (2011). 'Recognition as a Virtue in Social Work Practice.' *European Journal of Social Work*, 14, 2, 195–213.
Martin, R. and Barresi, J. (eds.) (2003). *Personal Identity*. Oxford: Blackwell Publishing.
McBeath, G. and Webb, S. (2002). 'Virtue Ethics and Social Work: Being Lucky, Realistic and not Doing one's Duty.' *British Journal of Social Work*, 32, 1015–36.
Okpych, N. and Yu, J. (2014). 'A Historical Analysis of Evidence-Based Practice in Social Work: The Unfinished Journey Toward an Empirically Grounded Profession.' *Social Service Review*, 88, 1, 3–58.

Pallisera, M., Fullana, J., Palaudarias, J.-M. and Badosa, M. (2013). 'Personal and Professional Development (or Use of Self) in Social Educator Training: An Experience Based on Reflective Learning.' *Social Work Education*, 32, 5, 576–89.
Parfit, D. (1984). *Reasons and Persons*. Oxford: Oxford University Press.
Parton, N. and O'Byrne, P. (2000). *Constructive Social Work: Towards a New Practice*. Basingstoke: Palgrave Macmillan.
Pavelová, L. (2014). 'Community Work or Community Social Work?' *Revista de Asistență Socială*, 13, 1, 7–15
Payne, M. (2005). *Modern Social Work Theory*. 3rd edn. New York: Lyceum Books.
Pierson, J. (2011). *Understanding Social Work: History and Context*. Maidenhead: Open University Press.
Reisch, M. and Andrews, J. (2002). *The Road Not Taken: A History of Radical Social Work in the United States*. London: Routledge.
Rudd, A. (2001). 'Reason and Ethics: MacIntyre and Kierkegaard.' In Davenport, J. and Rudd, A, (eds.), *Kierkegaard after MacIntyre: Essays on Freedom, Narrative and Virtue*. New York: Open Court Publishing, pp. 131–50.
Sayer, A. (2011). *Why Things Matter to People: Social Science, Values and Ethical Life*. Cambridge: Cambridge University Press.
Schram, S. (2000). *After Welfare: The Culture of Postindustrial Social Policy*. New York: New York University Press.
Sheldon, B. (2001). 'The Validity of Evidence-Based Practice in Social Work: A Reply to Stephen Webb.' *British Journal of Social Work*, 31, 801–9.
Specht, H. and Courtney, M. (1994). *Unfaithful Angels: How Social Work has Abandoned its Mission*. New York: The Free Press.
Stokes, P. (2008). 'Locke, Kierkegaard, and the Phenomenology of Personal Identity.' *International Journal of Philosophical Studies*, 16, 5, 645–72.
Taylor, C. (1985). *Philosophy and the Human Sciences*. Cambridge: Cambridge University Press.
—— (1989). *Sources of the Self*. Cambridge, MA: Harvard University Press.
—— (1991). *The Ethics of Authenticity*. Cambridge, MA: Harvard University Press.
—— (1994). 'The Politics of Recognition.' In Goldberg, D. (ed.), *Multiculturalism. A Critical Reader*. Oxford: Blackwell, pp. 25–73.
Vice, S. (2003). 'Literature and the Narrative Self.' *Philosophy*, 78, 1, 93–108.
Webb, S. (2001). 'Some Considerations on the Validity of Evidence-based Practice in Social Work.' *British Journal of Social Work*, 31, 57–79.

7
CULTURE
The culture industry

Turning (in)to culture

'Social space is now completely saturated with the image of culture', Fredric Jameson has claimed (Jameson 1998: 111). More than ever before, the very idea of 'the social' that creates and sustains the contexts for social work practice is mediated through 'the cultural'. In social work, this is visible in the increasingly broadening reaches of 'cultural competence' as part of its instruction. While originally focused on increasing awareness of racial and ethnic differences amongst service users, cultural competence can now refer to the complex layers of identity formation, and the multiple and overlapping strands of oppression, which social work deals with (see Rothman 2008). Since 2007, the NASW code of ethics has included the 'subjective experience' of a culture as part of cultural competence. In other words, rather than signifying the characteristics of a set of established group traditions over time, culture now also signifies individual actions and reactions. The more that cultures are recognised as distinguishable or different, and the more dispersed and decentred they seem to be in relation to dominant modes of thought and practice, the more important culture as a general term becomes to both. As such, Mike Featherstone points out that 'the more general decentring and fragmentation of culture has been accompanied by a recentring of culture' (1995: 3), within the study and knowledge-base of academics and practitioners alike.

> **Thinking through Practice**
>
> In what ways would you say your practice was engaged in or with 'culture', and how do you understand that term? Based on this, to what extent do you agree with Jameson's assertion that social space is 'saturated with the image of culture'?

The problem is that the term itself has become circulated so readily and with such vivacity that it has become a carrier of, or cipher for, an almost endless array of different interests, activities and agendas. Since the late 1960s, there have been 'cultural turns' not only in philosophy and the social sciences but also in global and local politics; not only in academic journals but also in the currents and trends of everyday social interactions; and, of course, it could well be said that there has been a cultural turn within culture itself. The recognition that culture is a mediator – if not *the* mediator – of thought and action, however, immediately gives rise to a tension between the local practices of any given culture (bracketing for the moment what this elusive term may actually mean or imply), and how this translates into a global or universal sense of values and knowledge. The dual attempt of organisations such as the International Federation of Social Work (IFSW) to hold both rigorous standards for social work practice across the globe, and to use such rigour as a force to challenge the global interconnection of oppression and marginalisation, must negotiate the question of culture.

It is important to frame this discussion in terms of two 'turns' to culture which underlie its emergence as a dominating concern for contemporary practice. The first turn stems from a fundamental paradox at the heart of globalisation. Globalisation, broadly conceived, signifies 'the intensification of worldwide social relations and interdependence' (Giddens 1998: 74). Polack affirms:

> In the new century, social work is confronted with a global system in which the world's people are bound together in a complex web of economic relationships. People's lives are now linked to lives of distant others through the clothes they wear, the energy that warms them and even the food they eat.
> (Polack 2004: 281)

This is not a problem in itself; after all, such economic relationships have been in existence since the Roman Empire at least. Even before this, Peter Sloterdijk argues that globalisation has been present since at least the ancient philosophers first began to conceive of the world as a rounded 'cosmos', and was perpetuated within the Enlightenment by the philosophical alignment of rationality and universality (Sloterdijk 2014: 8). And indeed, around 90 per cent of the world's trade is still carried on shipping routes that have remained similar since the sixteenth century. The recent relaxing of EU border controls with Romania and Bulgaria threatened (or so the right wing press claimed) to flood the United Kingdom with benefit-claiming criminals; a comparatively meagre number of migrants arrived. But whether explicitly or implicitly, the social work profession is nevertheless now always-already partaking in a global dialogue (see Parton 1996); however much the 'form and expression social work assumes in any particular place is locality specific and heterogeneous' (Dominelli 2010: 16).

Indeed, it is the rapid increase of global interconnectedness, travel and communication technologies, migration and markets and economic relations/effects that seems to erode the very boundaries of what may be considered 'locality specific'.

The adoption of specific policy programmes by institutions of global governance such as the European Union, World Trade Organisation, International Monetary Fund and World Bank means 'neoliberalism has fundamentally altered the conditions under which social work takes place and the conditions of life of service users' (Penna and O'Brien 2013: 138). Indeed, 'neoliberalism is now enshrined in global institutions that affect the domestic policy of all countries' (Penna and O'Brien 2013: 145). This erosion, however, is complicated by the paradoxical nature of globalisation itself. Economically, the more that the global economy develops its 'capacity to work as a unit in real time on a planetary scale' (Castells 1996: 92), the more inequalities seem to be produced. Lynne Healy (2008: 53) points out that while contemporary global reality is shaped by massive developments in science and technology, in spite of this – or maybe because of this – the number of poor, illiterate and unemployed people in the world continues to grow. Saskia Sassen has likewise questioned whether the growth of poverty in general is linked to the 'growth of an industrial complex oriented to the world market and significantly less dependent on local factors' (1991: 334). Such poverty is invariably articulated in terms of social categories (gender, age, communities etc.), which in turn bring to the fore signs and marks of 'culture'. Socially, meanwhile, the irony of globalisation is that the quicker our communication technologies enable information, goods and capital to traverse the world, the more differences between individuals are enhanced, and the more atomised communities seem to become. As conventional borders between groups dissolve, symbolic and imaginary borders – proliferated through 'cultural difference' – are required.

The second, and related, turn can be seen as a cultural turn within culture itself. This is the shift from what was, traditionally, seen as 'high culture' – art, aesthetics, opera, and so on – to 'low culture', which is the aesthetics of the everyday and the ordinary. While at first this seems only a tertiary issue to social work practice, in fact it is what happens to culture as an idea that in part contributes to the way in which the first problem is perceived. The achievement of this manifestation of the cultural turn was to recognise the value and worth of people's knowledge, actions and relations as worth celebrating and/or preserving, even if they lay outside of the traditional sphere of high culture. But this also broadens and renders far more complex the ways in which individuals not only carried multiple identities, but also suffered multiple forms of oppression which led them to become service users or social work clients. This confronted social workers with the problem of an 'equality of oppressions paradigm' (Razack and Jeffery 2002; Schiele 2007). The debate that followed was chiefly concerned with the extent to which the more traditional forms of cultural identification – what Charles Tilley (1999) termed the 'categorical inequalities' of gender, race and class – were dissipated by the broader interpretation of what constituted cultural practices, and, crucially, whether the enthusiasm of theorists to embrace such a levelling of oppression would leave social work students ill-prepared for the most widespread or deeply rooted forms of marginalisation.

If the first aspect concerned the relationship between the universal and the particular, the second is concerned with the centre at the margins. Given such complexities, it is not surprising that Culley notes, in the context of health research at

European or North American perspective: 'rather than look at the Third World at large', Spivak notes, we 'make everything identical with the problem at home' (1990: 64).

This relation of opposition is fundamental to the way in which systems of knowledge from the West have framed the 'other' of culture. We have seen why culture emerges as a significant condition of understanding the world through the processes of globalisation. But modern globalisation is, itself, embedded within further histories of colonialism that also frame the way that culture emerges *as important*. Hence Spivak notes how the 'real difficulty with cultural politics' is the tendency to re-assert 'old attitudes disguised in one way or another' (1990: 64).

The sense in which the 'other' is formed as a mirror image of the self is rooted in the dualisms of modern philosophy. As we have seen in the last two chapters, the Western sense of self is characterised by a repudiation of the non-self, and the various forms that threaten the uniqueness of the individual who reasons for themselves: the traditional, the irrational, the heteronomous and so on. That which is 'other' is, then, both seen as powerful (as a threat to the modern, Western conception of the individual) at the same time as it is necessarily subordinate to the self. The rise of culture as a particular formation of the 'other' finds its strongest expression within the orientalism of the nineteenth century. In his famous work, Edward Said (1978) argued that orientalism was not only an academic tradition of study, teaching and writing about the orient (which typically signified anything 'east' of Europe); it was also a style of thought based upon the ontological and epistemological distinction made between the 'orient' and (usually) the 'occident'. Key to this distinction was a political purpose, in which orientalism served as a Western approach for the domination and restructuring of the orient. In his wide-ranging study, Said suggests that representations of the 'other' serve both 'to characterise the orient as alien and to incorporate it schematically on a theatrical stage whose audience, manager and actors are for Europe' (1978: 71). The fascination with the orient that overtook the European intelligentsia of the time served, correspondingly, to mark out a core identity of 'the West' which was otherwise under challenge or lacking. At a time when urban poverty was becoming increasingly problematic in Europe, images of rural destitution within archaic feudal kingdoms were sent back from the orient. At a time when sexual morality was increasingly scrutinised and regulated within the European middle classes, images of lavish and seductive cultures of polygamy and harems represented the colonies. Europe's colonial ambitions were legitimised on both an assertion of dominance – Europe was more developed and 'modernised' than the primitive colonies – and an inherent desire, not just for wealth, but for that which Europe had perceived itself to have 'lost' within the process of modernity.[1]

Such representations of the 'other' were not limited to colonial ambition, however. Modern European philosophy has historically concerned itself with 'universal' knowledge and approaches (think of Kant's categorical imperative, or, indeed, the principles of modern science itself): it is built around the need to *transcend* specific and local situations. This lends itself to particular formations of both systemic 'truth' and pragmatic 'effectiveness'. The positing of alternatives to European thought – the 'indigenous' knowledge of the other – has traditionally been figured in opposition to the 'mythical' and 'folklore' of the non-European. In short, 'culture' is local, and in being irredeemably local, opposes universal 'knowledge'.

If the age of colonial empires is now in the past, their legacy on the way we articulate cultural difference is still very much in effect in the 'postcolonial' era. As Payne and Askeland note, globalisation 'draws attention to, confirms and increases postcolonial inequalities' (2008: 59), specifically in terms of education and the structures of social care provision. Concerns for the way in which global social work agendas have pursued the same 'modernising' techniques of colonialism – techniques which remain inherent to the neo-liberal agenda within globalisation – are characterised in Midgely's (2001) concept of 'professional imperialism'. Just as colonial powers advanced into their territories through the force not just of physical power, but also epistemological and technological dominance, so too Midgely sees the advance of 'professionalised social work' as transferring, in a unidirectional way, European and North American 'expertise' to poorer countries; countries which often have no previous tradition or history of these particular standards of the 'profession'. Indeed, for Wehbi, this follows a 'colonial construction' whereby poorer nations are represented 'as inferior and in need of saving', which in turn 'have been crucial in maintaining Northern influence within international relations and to justify historical and contemporary imperialistic practices' (Wehbi 2011: 27). By assuming superior expertise on the basis of technological and economic successes, Western social workers re-articulate the colonialist initiative.

These concerns have been voiced not only in terms of the development of recognisable social work roles and institutions in former colonies, but also in the very idea of a unified 'international social work' agenda. Hence, Erika Haug has wondered 'how we can speak of social work's role in promoting global social justice, without first acknowledging social work's shadow role in the perpetuation of injustice in the form of the colonialist project that has dismissed and displaced countless cultural systems around the world' (2005: 127). Indeed, if the dominant model of professionalisation arose in response to the industrialisation of Europe and the United States (see Weiss-Gal and Welbourne 2008: 282), in the case of the expansion of professional social work across the globe, then 'exporting' social care practices can be complicit with *driving* industrialisation. Hence, Midgely argues that the kind of 'expertise' that travelled from the 'developed' nations to poorer ones was directed towards particular organisational consistency. In other words, it is an expertise which reflects the ideals of Western consumerism; what Ritzer (1993) famously termed the 'MacDonaldisation' of society, whereby everyday practice is regulated by the key principles of efficiency, calculability, uniformity that arise from the fast-food industry rather than social care; on the grounds that this 'massive bureaucratisation of everyday life' results in progressive standardisation (Featherstone 1995: 8).

Both Ritzer and Midgely's cases have been contested. Closer examination of how each nation has adopted social care and social work reveals far more nuanced interrelations between former colonies and European powers, such as a with the reconceptualisation movement in South American social work (see Healy 2008: 155–6); in much the same way as a closer examination of MacDonald's restaurants shows a complex development of restaurants responding to local contexts (see Miller and McHoul 1998), in a manner that Robertson (1995) described as 'glocalisation' or cultural hybridity. But it remains the case that the issue of postcolonialism can operate in both obvious and subtle ways. For example, Payne and Askeland point out that:

> Social work education is in a global market. Those who have the resources to produce and market social work literature and academic courses are able to disseminate their social work theory and practice throughout the world as preferred or unique professional ways of handling social issues. In doing so, they ignore the differences between local contexts in which their knowledge is produced and those where it is used. (2008: 59)

The range of 'postcolonial' critiques (such as Said 1978, Spivak 1990 and Bhabha 1994) challenges this hegemonic approach to the 'othering' of culture. The postcolonial critique, however, does not simply argue for a reversal or resistance to the cultural dominance of certain symbols – efficiency, uniformity, calculability – of 'good practice.' For such imperialism instates a dichotomy between the 'expert' nations and the 'folk' localities which they aim to transform, modernise, and bring into the 'global' standards of social work. Criticising the latent imperialism of organisations such as the IFSW by appealing to some kind of fixed, inherently worthy or essential local practice in fact only reasserts this same dichotomy. It maintains the *temporality* of the colonial: the 'idea of time as a progressive, ordered whole' (Bhabha 1994: 59). It is not, as the work of Fanon argued, a question of political rights (which assumes a universalist liberalism), or of ontological identity (that is: 'what is this culture? Who is 'cultural'?). Rather, 'there is no master narrative or realist perspective that provides a background of social and historical facts' for a subject or group that is 'historicised in the heterogeneous assemblage of the texts of history, literature, science, myth' (Bhabha 1994: 59). In other words, postcolonial thought begins from the sense that 'culture' is a practice that is both deeply historical, but never as the subject of its history:

> The colonial subject is always 'overdetermined from without', Fanon writes. It is through image and fantasy – those orders that figure transgressively on the borders of history and the unconscious – that Fanon most profoundly evokes the colonial condition. (Bhabha 1994: 59)

This over-determination is often obscured, however, because what is recognised and valued within a 'local culture' is typically the precise opposite of the global culture. Local culture is typically seen as a small and boundaried space, premised on face-to-face habits and practices that, by virtue of these 'habits', is knowable only through the lived experience of 'being there'. For example, Dominelli speaks glowingly of how 'indigenous knowledge is noted for the connections it makes between people and their physical environment and the reverence with which the physical sphere is regarded' (Dominelli 2010: 120).

Thinking through Practice

Dominelli cites approvingly Tait-Rolleston and Pehi-Barlow's article on 'A Maori Social Work Construct' (2001), which recounts how the indigenous Maori understanding of the world as inherently spiritual, interrelating notions of kinship, family, genealogy and the land, allows Maori communities to survive the 'brutal treatment' (Dominelli 2010: 123) of both historical colonial practices, and its present-day incarnation in the form of disproportionate numbers of interventions made by both police and social care authorities. 'This indigenous approach', Dominelli writes of Maori social work strategies based on the Family Group Conference method of intervention, 'contrasts starkly with the less visionary and fragmented approaches currently being adopted in the West' (123).

The work of theorists such as Toon van Meijl has raised the complexity of the Maori position, however, specifically in terms of the way in which cultural aspects of identity are 'rephrased' and 'reconstituted' (rather than simply remembered or called upon) in the light of post-colonial revivals of indigenous traditions. Noting how the relevance of such traditions emerges predominantly at points where access to economic and political resources is unequal, he argues that the 'reconstitution of culture and the renaissance of traditional symbols of ethnicity cannot be considered in isolation of the context in which the competition for resources takes place' (van Meijl 2004: 6).

In what ways do you think that the Maori subject – the case of a young male offender from a Maori community, for example – is 'overdetermined from without' in Dominelli's argument?

Featherstone notes that this 'sense of belonging, the common sedimented experiences and cultural forms which are associated with a place, is crucial to the concept of a local culture' (Featherstone 1995: 92). But any such drawing of boundaries is, he continues, a *relational* act 'which depends upon the figuration of significant other localities within which one seeks to situate it' (1995: 92). Appealing to a cultural identity as 'local' demands a comparative site whether a different locality, such as a comparison between different areas of a city defined by the ethnicity of their inhabitants, or a broader global comparison, whereby specific articulations of culture are marked out as different from the universalist pretensions of modern liberalism. When such a site is articulated as a sense of 'cultural heritage' – whether this is a shared history, a shared form of life-philosophy (as Dominelli suggests), a language, a cuisine, a dress – it is necessary to question the grounds on which these relational acts are performed, and where they appear. Indeed, as Nostra (2005) argues, the conservation of heritage can be positioned as an opposing force to globalising economic development. But in this light, once we step outside our delight with Dominelli's holistic indigeneity, we may feel some worry: first, that it risks a certain exoticising or even fetishising 'indigenous knowledge' as exhibiting a form of essential, yet primitive, ecological form of care;

second, that the corollary to such appreciation is raw forms of fundamentalism: that is, a sense of culture premised on the threat of its disappearance, or a nostalgic yearning for that which has never quite existed.

For this reason, Bhabha warns that the 'postcolonial perspective resists the attempt at holistic forms of social explanation. It forces a recognition of the more complex cultural and political boundaries that exist on the cusp of these often opposed political spheres' (Bhabha 1994: 248). In contrast to Dominelli's account, then, for Bhabha postcolonial critique forces us 'to rethink the profound limitations of a consensual and collusive "liberal" sense of cultural community. It insists that cultural and political identity are constructed through a *process* of alterity' rather than an affirmation of existing dichotomies. Indeed, Bhabha argues that 'the time for "assimilating" minorities to holistic and organic notions of cultural value has dramatically passed' (251).

Culture as a production: the culture industry

Such a rethinking is not necessarily a clear and uplifting appeal to alternative viewpoints. The postcolonial theorist Gayatri Spivak, for example, renounces the idea that any such discourse can separate itself from the structures that inform its production. Understanding that cultural identity is constructed is, for Spivak, only half the story: construction implies the possibilities of deconstruction; but this play in and around the nature of alterity does not lend itself to any kind of immediate 'politics', as we saw in Chapter 6. The postcolonial critique thus leaves some uncomfortable questions for those wanting to uphold the prominence of 'locality' to social work practice; as this requires theorising 'locality' in a way which negotiates the complex relations between identity, alterity and power that produce our sense of culture. For example, Badiou, following Deleuze, argues that it is capitalism which 'demands a permanent creation of subjective and territorial identities in order for its principle of movement to homogenize its space of action. [...] the capitalist logic of the general equivalent and the identitarian and cultural logic of communities or minorities form an articulate whole' (Badiou 2003: 10–11). In short: capitalism *wants* us to be cultural.

Such an argument was originally put forward by Theodore Adorno and his longtime collaborator Max Horkheimer, in their thesis on the 'culture industry', which first appeared in their book on the *Dialectic of Enlightenment*. For Adorno, the problem of 'culture' was not rooted in indigenous practices, ethnic identities or postcolonial others, but rather it was about the massification of entertainment, and the retreat of distinctions between 'high culture' and 'low culture'. While this may, at first, appear to be a completely separate realm from our discussion thus far, it is also the case that both culture as an essence and culture as an 'other' were fundamentally *mediated*: whether through the culturalisation of politics, or the historical conditions of colonialism. Adorno's attention is on the media themselves, and the way that they *produce* cultural phenomena. Whereas our earlier discussion mapped out the ways in which cultural identity was differentiated as 'essential', Adorno and Horkheimer's critique probes into the workings of the images, symbols and words around us that perpetuate not only the idea of what culture 'is' (or what it is to be 'cultural'), but also what alternative conceptions there may be.

By the culture industry, then, they do not mean a literal industry producing culture, but rather the standardisation and 'rationalisation of distribution techniques' (1991: 100) that cultural objects and practices are subject to. In this sense, Adorno's thesis links the active creation of highly stereotyped and homogeneous cultural forms that provide the masses with a limited number of models of lifestyle, behaviours and identity, and with a uniform set of values. Focusing on society in the US, Adorno argues that the 'free pursuits' of leisure and entertainment were subject to the monopolisation of powerful interest groups. In this sense, people's lives away from work were as subject to regulation and control as when they were at work. If the likes of Said note that culture becomes distinctive as an 'other' in the nineteenth century, Adorno and Horkheimer suggest that culture becomes absorbed into the everyday through the proliferation of the mass media: 'All forms of everyday knowledge, understanding and communication are effectively controlled by the overarching system of bureaucratic and administrative control through which organised capitalism is managed and maintained' (Bennett 2005: 18).

> The effectiveness of the culture industry was not secured through a deceptive ideology, but by the removal from the consciousness of the masses of any alternative to capitalism. The dominant culture of late capitalism served to promote the repression of all forms of conflict, heterogeneity and particularity from the cultural sphere. (Stevenson 1995: 53)

Culture lost its power of separation from the lived experience of the everyday. Adorno argued that, before the advent of mass media, 'culture, in the true sense, did not simply accommodate itself to human beings; but it always simultaneously raised a protest against the petrified relations under which they lived'. However, once 'culture becomes wholly assimilated to and integrated in those petrified relations, human beings are once more debased' (Adorno 1991: 100). Culture becomes fetishised into particular objects, signs and symbols; but in doing so, the production of culture *itself* becomes faceless and omnipresent. And hence our opening quote from Jameson: social space becomes saturated with images of culture, but robbed of its practical, interactive and context-specific values which would give it a meaning above any other.

Thinking through Practice

Earlier, we saw Johnson and Munch claim that cultural competence in social work education provided 'concrete information on [...] practices of various cultural groups' which helped to 'alleviate social workers' level of anxiety about attempting to grasp myriad, ever-changing cultures' (2009: 224).

> In his essay 'Culture Industry Reconsidered', Adorno argues that:
>
> > In a supposedly chaotic world [the culture industry] provides human beings with something like standards for orientation, and that alone seems worthy of approval. However, what its defenders imagine is preserved by the culture industry is in fact all the more thoroughly destroyed by it. (Adorno 1991: 103)
>
> The appeal to order alone is not a mark of 'culture', for Adorno, because culture itself attempted 'to maintain a grasp on the good life' (104), rather than mere convention or order.
>
> What are the differences, then, between what Adorno describes as the culture industry, and the models of cultural competence critiqued by Johnson and Munch? Is it simply the form they take – mass media on the one hand, and education programmes on the other – or is there something more significant separating them?

Despite the deep suspicion of the media amongst many social work professionals – and what Chenot (2011) refers to as the 'vicious cycle' of negative images of social work passed around media and governments alike – Adorno's vision of the mass media may seem quaintly limited. If the media forms of the 1950s were a relatively cohesive, didactic body, the range of contemporary 'social' media depends upon user participation as much as it does the 'political propaganda' Adorno feared. Rather than the media acting as a didactic instrument of the powerful political or corporate elite, van Dijk suggests that 'it can be said that their common ideologies are jointly produced, each acting within its own sphere of influence and control, but each also dependent on the other' (1995: 29). The emergence of user-created media forms suggests a potential to re-frame the ways in which cultural differences are communicated. As Gianni Vattimo suggests, the success of the increasing number of cultural forms that 'liberate social minorities that previously had no voice' (2004: 125) cannot be ignored, and this may make Adorno's view on the use of culture industry now seem unduly pessimistic. Initiatives both large and small – from UNESCO's International Programme for the Development of Communication (IPDC), to projects such as the Zhoriben.net social networking site, established for members of the Roma community across Europe – have aimed to promote distinctive cultural identities within the context of globalised media. What remains from Adorno's critique, I think, is the problem of how to assert that certain cultural forms or expressions should be recognised as more *significant* than others: how the use of social media for promoting the voices of minorities, and challenging dominant ideas of what constitutes 'cultural practice', is prioritised over those that do not.

This is not a question of cultural form, but cultural hermeneutics. In this sense, Adorno's critique suffers less from his account of media itself, and more for precisely the same reason that Said's concept of Orientalism has been harshly criticised (see

Mellor 2004). That is, in criticising the dissolution of everything into 'culture', it fails to account for any sense of self-reflexivity on the part of the individuals within the cultural relationship. Johnson and Munch have alerted us to the fact that we cannot simply engage with 'culture' on a face-to-face level without attending to the epistemological commitments we are making. At the same time, while the historical, material and conceptual conditions of engaging with 'culture' are at work, it is important not to overlook the 'indigenous context' (Gray and Fook 2004) in which such conditions are actually encountered. While the colonial practices which frame culture take place across symbolic, aesthetic and experiential forms, this does not mean that 'living' culture is itself abstract or anonymous. In fact, it is precisely because the colonialist subjugation and marginalisation the 'culture industry' produces is *not* an abstract system – because economic and cultural operations are real – that the possibility remains for articulating ways in which this depoliticising can be countered.

Adorno's major contribution to the discussion of culture is to question where, given the extent to which cultural forms saturate our experience, we can sensibly draw a line between the essentialist a priori categories of 'the cultural' and the a posteriori experiences of culture – or even whether such a line can be drawn. Thinking about cultural difference affirmatively and positively is not achieved through the simple appeal to 'lived experience' – as any such experience is always mediated, historicised, and even hybridised. Instead, it is a case of appealing to a reflexive and lived *interpretation*.

Culture and the interpretation of local practice

Being aware of how culture as a term becomes recognisable and significant allows us to think through ways of avoiding Adorno's (and, to a lesser extent, Said's) pessimism about the visibility of cultural significance as reductive or damaging to the content of culture itself. Negotiating the complexities of colonialism as a medium brings to light the ways in which culture is a reflexive and interpretative activity. Hence, against the vision of culture as an ordering or regulating function (as with Adorno and, again, to a lesser extent with Said) Michel de Certeau argued that 'if culture is really going to exist, it is not enough to be the author of social practices; these social practices need to have meaning for those who effectuate them' (1997: 67).

This is not a case of simply re-inserting 'agency' into the discussion, in a way that repeats the Enlightenment separation of 'self' from 'tradition' by insisting on 'agency' outside or against 'cultural influence'. To the extent that culture *means* something (that is, to the extent that it is formed through heritage, locality, narrative etc.), rather than being an arbitrary or contingent act or expression, it must be situated within a context of interest, involving some kind of exchange, appropriation or transformation of its social space. It is from such interests that the 'agency' of culture emerges.

Such interests can be both positive and negative. A sense of shared identity based on meaningful social practices – whether we term these 'traditions', 'cultures' or something else – is key to successful interpretation, which, as we saw in Chapter 1, Gadamer's hermeneutics begins to sketch out. Lynne Healy (2008: 291–2) recounts a case study in which a six-year-old Hispanic girl is referred to a child protection agency, at risk of neglect. The child had suffered a rash, but despite advice from a school nurse, the mother had not consulted a doctor. When asked about the situation at home by a social worker, the child would say nothing. When the social worker visited the home, the mother would also be reluctant to provide basic information. When the child welfare supervisor (who was of Peruvian descent) went to visit the family, she realised – from her language and appearance – that the family were South American illegal residents; hence the mother would not visit a doctor, and the child would not speak of their situation at school. From this shift in the interpretative relationship between worker and family, she was able to offer support for the child. While it is easy to focus, in this case, on the actions at work – the referral, the visit, the outcomes – it is also true to say that what shifts between the charge of neglect and the location of support is an interpretative awareness. By recognising, and reconfiguring, the interest and purposiveness of the 'cultural context', the agency of the individuals emerged.

Likewise, articulating the interests of a 'cultural interaction' can be a strong basis for resistant practice. An example of this is Carmen Lavoie's empirical study of community organisation aimed at addressing racialised oppression in Quebec. Lavoie notes that, broadly construed, 'neighborhood community organizing practice predominantly constructed issues of race as issues of individual difference and need' (2012: 250). The ideas voiced by practitioners of the need to be 'open' to minority culture in order to best 'help' them carry a number of distinct 'discursive functions' that affect the staging of culture within the practice itself: 'being open' not only reflects the values of a liberal, pluralist society, it also assumes the capacity for practitioners to be 'open' or 'neutral'; it supposes that any assumptions the practitioners have are discoverable rather than deeply rooted; and it assumes that 'community organizers and residents enter into any exchange as equals' (248). While appearing to be something of a natural position to engage with 'cultural difference', Lavoie concludes that 'such approaches signal an individual-level analysis and contribute to a discourse of neutrality that places inequality and injustice on the basis of race outside the scope of change' (250). Against such neutrality, however, re-examining the *purposiveness* with which the community organisation practices approached 'culture' allowed alternative accounts to emerge that politicised, rather than accepted, the everyday experience of racial marginalisation. By constructing residents 'as agents and as people situated within a set of historical, political, and social conditions that contribute to inequality and oppression' (251), practitioners were able to highlight the conflicts between a sense of 'Canadian' culture as open and tolerant, and the country's history of oppression and treatment of minorities. As Lavoie quotes one practitioner: 'The problem is not because the immigrants have a different culture. The problem is that we all have culture, including people from here, and the fact that it is not neutral the way you work' (253).

What this example shows is how speaking from a cultural perspective opens up the relational aspect of any shared social practice. In both Healy's and Lavoie's very different examples, the aspects we identify as 'cultural' are specific to the interests and meaning of the relationships involved. In the case of the community workers in Quebec, this appeared from the task of articulating the contradictions between social care and the treatment of minorities, whereby particular forms of practice were framed as cultural that would otherwise not be. In the case of the Peruvian child welfare supervisor, a shared investment in cultural heritage allowed an otherwise hidden cultural dimension to the initial assessment – the inexistence of the illegal resident – to be heard, and for the specific problems of the family to thus be addressed.

In this sense, interpretations of, or narratives from, individual experiences can be as much about repairing or giving coherence to a fragmented cultural heritage as they are representative of a fixed, core 'essence' (see Irving and Young 2004: 220). Affirming a particular cultural standpoint as significant will always carry the risk of producing (or reproducing) a form of the 'culture industry'. At the same time, what remains fundamental to social work within cross-cultural contexts is its relational core. In this sense, the question, then, is not about what culture is, but in what senses culture is important to a particular relationship *at a given time*: for example, the relationship between social worker and immigrant child being re-housed with extended family; or the relationship between the child and the family; the relationship between the family and their sense of migrant identity, and so on. It is perhaps in this sense that Healy (2008) recommends that a dialogical approach, carried in particular through the exchange of knowledge and education, rather than a corrective one, is the best strategy for cross-cultural difference: 'learning from' rather than 'knowing about'.

This may, however, overlook the inherent antagonism that often accompanies cultural differences. 'Increasingly,' Bhabha notes, 'the issue of cultural difference emerges at points of social crises, and the questions of identity that it raises are agonistic' (1994: 254). This agonistic sense is not necessarily outright conflict – wherein the 'just' or 'right' or 'powerful' immediately gain an upper hand in deciding the outcome – but rather a problem of what Charles Taylor terms incommensurability. Cultural practices such as approaches to disciplining children, the use of 'traditional' healing practices or hierarchical decision-making structures within families – all conventional markers of a displaced colonial 'culture' – are clearly not identical to the countervailing orthodoxies of Western, liberal society, but neither are they necessarily *separate*: in Taylor's words, 'they are different, yet they somehow occupy the same space' (1985: 145). In such cases, this *requires* a judgement to be made. But given the risks involved with identifying culture that we have discussed, on what basis might a judgement be made, beyond the recognition of the historical conditions of cultural identity?

Taylor proposes that we look for a 'minimal rationality' that allows us to compare, contrast, argue and make transcultural judgements without ethnocentrism. Rationality is, however – as we saw in the previous chapter – not a formal sense of reasoning, but rather the 'human activities of articulation which give the value of rationality its sense' (151). Culture is no longer an epistemological function, but an enunciative practice (Bhabha 1994: 254). In this sense, competing cultures will both articulate 'different features of the world in some perspicuous order' (Taylor 1985: 150). They are both forms of rationality, in this sense, but Taylor argues that at least in some senses one can lay claim to a more effective rationality than the other, if its articulation 'commands the attention' of the other by achieving 'a more perspicuous order'. To take the relativist stance against this – that one man's terrorist is another's freedom fighter, or one parent's neglect is another's spiritual healing – merely re-imposes an essentialist sense of culture which ignores the agonistic context in which culture emerges in its contemporary form. To take the less extreme, but no less valid, stance that warns against the latent possibility of re-inscribing imperialist practices under the guise of 'perspicuous order' – as many of the critiques of 'Professional Imperialism', or of the universality of Human Rights have done, for example – is to some extent a necessary wariness.

The key is the extent to which this can be said to 'make sense'. As Weiss-Gal and Welbourne note in their comparative study of international social work, certain professional features were common to all of those countries: 'the establishment of professional organisations, the formulation or adoption of a professional code of ethics, the development and dissemination of a specific body of knowledge (although to varying extents), and the placement of social work training in institutions of higher education' (2008: 288). However, other features of 'professionalism' were largely absent in areas such as licensing practice, protected titles, and monopolies over the field of practice. Could it be argued that in such countries, these rationalities of professionalism simply make less sense? Do they make less 'perspicuous order' than their application in the US or the UK? It seems entirely possible to note this; as Webb (2003) notes, any structurally transformative project on a global level for social work is only ever filtered and applied through local and reflexive cultural practice.

But noting these differences does not preclude critique, or imply a simplistic referral to 'what happens here'. Culture, above all, has to make sense, and this is a double-edge remit: on the one hand, any global social work agenda has to be grounded in concrete and realistic objectives 'wherein social work has a proven track record' (Webb 2003). Practice is always 'encumbered by local practice and experience'. But this is not its *epistemological* foundation; it is rather the way in which knowledge and theory are articulated meaningfully. On the other hand, this requirement for meaningfulness is a demand. Appeals to 'cultural sensitivity' must form part of a virtuous hermeneutic circle, aware of the historical, material and narrative context within which 'culture' is articulated.

Thinking through Practice

Writing of the possibility of global social work agendas, Erika Haug argues that 'by focusing on common goals and values such as a clear commitment to human rights and social justice, rather than buy in to a Western 'scientific' 'professional' knowledge base, more space is created for diverse expressions of social work from around the world to be included in the International Social Work conversation' (2005: 132).

Is this a similar approach, do you think, to Taylor's 'minimal rationality'? How does such a commitment shape the way in which 'culture' appears as a set of practices within social work?

Note

1   The same argument has applied to the notion of an 'underclass' amongst the poor within Western societies – prominent not only in nineteenth century Europe (see McClintock 1995), but also in the United States in the 1980s (see Murray 1996) and still today (see Jones 2011) – that forms a dyadic opposition to the values of the better off, morally competent middle classes: laziness, moral ineptitude and lack of aspiration are cited as cultural aspects of social inequalities, which reproduces in clear terms the language of colonialism (see Sennett 2012: 3–33).

References

Abrams, L. and Moio, J. (2009). 'Critical Race Theory and the Cultural Competence Dilemma in Social Work Education.' *Journal of Social Work Education*, 45, 2, 245–61.
Adorno, T. (1991). *The Culture Industry*. London: Routledge.
Adorno, T. and Horkheimer, M. (1997 [1947]). *Dialectic of Enlightenment*. London: Verso.
Badiou, A. (2001). *Ethics: An Essay on the Understanding of Evil*. P. Hallward (trans.). London: Verso.
—— (2003). *Saint Paul: The Foundation of Universalism*. R. Brassier (trans.). Stanford, CA: Stanford University Press
Baudrillard, J. (2002). *The Singular Objects of Architecture*. Minneapolis, MN: University of Minnesota Press.
Bennett, A. (2005). *Culture and Everyday Life*. London: Sage.
Bhabha, H. (1994). *The Location of Culture*. London: Routledge.
Brown, W. (2006). *Regulating Aversion: Tolerance in the Age of Identity and Empire*. Princeton, NJ: Princeton University Press.
Castells, M. (1996). *The Rise of Network Society*. Oxford: Blackwell.
Chenot, D. (2011). 'The Vicious Cycle: Recurrent Interactions among the Media, Politicians, the Public, and Child Welfare Services Organizations.' *Journal of Public Child Welfare*, 5, 2, 167–84.
Culley, L. (2000). 'Working with Diversity: Beyond the Factfile.' In Davies, C., Finlay, L. and Bullman, A. (eds), *Changing Practice in Health and Social Care*. London: Sage, pp. 131–42.
De Certeau, M. (1997). *Culture in the Plural*. T. Conley (trans.). Minneapolis, MN: University of Minnesota Press.
Dominelli, L. (2010). *Social Work in a Globalizing World*. Cambridge: Polity Press.
Fanon, F. (1986). *Black Skin, White Masks*. London: Pluto.
Featherstone, M. (1995). *Undoing Culture: Globalization, Postmodernism and Identity*. London: Sage.
Giddens, A. (1998). *The Third Way: the Renewal of Social Democracy*. Cambridge: Polity.
Gray, M. and Fook, J. (2004). 'The Quest for a Universal Social Work: Some Issues and Implications.' *Social Work Education*, 23, 5, 635–44.
Green, R., Kiernan-Stern, M. and Baskind, F. (2005). 'White Social Workers' Attitudes about People of Color.' *Journal of Ethnic & Cultural Diversity in Social Work*, 14, 1, 47–68.
Haug, E. (2005). 'Critical reflections on the emerging discourse of international social work.' *International Social Work*, 48, 2, 126–35.
Healy, L. (2008). *International Social Work: Professional Action in an Interdependent World*. 2nd edn. Oxford: Oxford University Press.
Irving, A. and Tomas Young, T. (2004). '"Perpetual Liminality": Re-Readings of Subjectivity and Diversity in Clinical Social Work Classrooms.' *Smith College Studies in Social Work*, 74, 2, 213–27.
Jameson, F. (1998). *The Cultural Turn: Selected Writings on the Postmodern, 1983–1998*. London: Verso.

Johnson, L. and Munch, S. (2009). 'Fundamental Contradictions in Cultural Competence.' *Social Work*, 54, 3, 220–31.
Jones, O. (2011). *Chavs: the Demonization of the Working Class*. London: Verso.
Lavoie, C. (2012). 'Race, Power and Social Action in Neighborhood Community Organizing: Reproducing and Resisting the Social Construction of the Other.' *Journal of Community Practice*, 20, 241–59.
Lawrence, K. (2001). 'Expanding Comprehensiveness: Structural Racism and Community Building in the United States.' In Pierson, J. and Smith, J. (eds.), *Rebuilding Community: Policy and Practice*. Basingstoke: Palgrave Macmillan, pp. 34–63.
McClintock, A. (1995). *Imperial Leather: Race, Gender and Sexuality in the Colonial Conquest*. London: Routledge.
Mellor, P. (2004). 'Orientalism, Representation and Religion: the Reality behind the Myth', *Religion*, 34, 99–112.
Midgely, J. (2001) 'The Critical Perspective in Social Development.' *Social Development Issues*, 23, 1, 42–50.
Miller, T. and McHoul, A. (1998). *Popular Culture and Everyday Life*. London: Sage.
Murray, C. (1996). *Charles Murray and the Underclass: The Developing Debate*. London: Civitas.
Nostra, E. (2005). *Cultural Heritage and Sustainable Economic and Social Development*. Belgium: European Cultural Heritage Forum.
Park, Y. (2005). 'Culture as Deficit: A Critical Discourse Analysis of the Concept of Culture in Contemporary Social Work Discourse.' *Journal of Sociology and Social Welfare*, 32, 11–33.
Parton, N. (1996) (ed.) *Social Theory, Social Change and Social Work*. London: Routledge.
Payne, M. and Askeland, G. (2008). *Globalization and International Social Work: Postmodern Change and Challenge*. Farnham: Ashgate Publishing.
Penna, S. and O'Brien, M. (2013). 'Neoliberalism.' In Gray, M. and Webb, S. (eds.), *Social Work Theories and Methods*. 2nd edn. London: Sage.
Polack, R. (2004). 'Social Justice and the Global Economy: New Challenges for Social Work in the 21st Century.' *Social Work*, 49, 2, 261–90.
Razack, N. and Jeffery, D. (2002). 'Critical Race Discourse and Tenets for Social Work.' Canadian Social Work Review, 19, 2, 257–71.
Ritzer, G. (1993). *The McDonaldization of Society*. London: Sage.
Robertson, R. (1995). 'Glocalization: Time-Space and Homogeneity-Heterogeneity.' In Featherstone, M., Lash, S. and Robertson, R. (eds), *Global Modernities*. London: Sage, pp. 25–44.
Rothman (2008). *Cultural Competence in Process and Practice: Building Bridges*. Boston, MA: Pearson Education.
Said, E. (1978). *Orientalism*. London: Vintage Books.
Sassen, S. (1991). *The Global City: New York, London, Tokyo*. Princeton, NJ: Princeton University Press.
Schiele, J. H. (2007). 'Implications of the Equality-of-Oppressions Paradigm for Curriculum Content on People of Color.' *Journal of Social Work Education*, 43, 83–100.
Sennett, R. (2012). *Together: The Rituals, Pleasures and Politics of Cooperation*. London: Penguin.
Sloterdijk, P. (2014). *In the World Interior of Capital*. W. Hoban (trans.). Cambridge: Polity.
Spivak, G. (1990). *The Post-Colonial Critic: Interviews, Strategies, Dialogues*. London: Routledge.
Stevenson, N. (1995). *Understanding Media Cultures*. London: Sage.
Taylor, C. (1985). *Philosophy and the Human Sciences*. Cambridge: Cambridge University Press.
Tilley, C. (1999). *Durable Inequality*. Irvine, CA: University of California Press.
Van Dijk, T. (1995). 'Power and the News Media.' In Paletz, D. (ed.), *Political Communication and Action*. Cresskill, NJ: Hampton Press, pp. 9–36.

Van Meijl, T. (2004). 'Introduction.' In van Meijl, T. and Miedema, J. (eds.), *Shifting Images of Identity in the Pacific*. Leiden: KITLV Press, pp. 1–19.

Van Ufford, P. (1996). 'Reality Exists: Acknowledging the Limits of Active and Reflexive Anthropological Knowledge.' In van Harskamp, A. (ed.), *Conflicts in Social Science*. London: Routledge, pp. 22–43.

Vattimo, G. (2004). *Nihilism and Emancipation: Ethics, Politics and Law*. New York: Columbia University Press.

Webb, S. (2003). 'Local Orders and Global Chaos in Social Work.' *European Journal of Social Work*, 6, 2, 191–204.

Wehbi, S. (2011). 'Key Theoretical Concepts for Teaching International Social Work.' *Social Work Review*, 10, 4, 23–9.

Weiss-Gal, I. and Welbourne, P. (2008). 'The Professionalisation of Social Work: A Cross-National Exploration.' *International Journal of Social Welfare*, 17, 281–90.

Williams, C. (2006). 'The Epistemology of Cultural Competence.' *Families in Society: The Journal of Contemporary Social Services*, 87, 209–20.

Žižek, S. (2009). *Violence*. London: Verso.

8
KNOWLEDGE

Professionalised practice and the locus of expertise

The locus of expertise

Throughout this book I have been outlining the ways in which the concerns of philosophy – and in particular the concerns of philosophy as a form of cultural hermeneutics – resonate with debates within social work itself. In this final chapter, I want to draw some of these observations together under the question of expertise. In many ways, the themes that this question raises bring us full circle to the book's opening discussion, as they revolve around the centrality of 'practice-wisdom' as an interpretative activity, and in particular its relationship to the idea of social work as a 'profession'. As such, I want to conclude the book here with just a few, rather schematic points, regarding the ground on which such interpretative expertise stands, before re-considering the relationship between social work and philosophy in this light.

When we ask what kind of expertise social workers should have, on what basis they hold expertise, how this expertise is demonstrated, and how it might be challenged, these questions are not fully answered by simply referring to descriptive standards for qualification, capabilities frameworks, educational curricula and so on. While these show what social workers should *know* and *do*, and what they should be able to do, the question of expertise instead concerns the 'where' and the 'how' of knowledge, not just the 'what'.

> **Thinking through Practice**
>
> What is the difference between knowledge and expertise, in your view? Think about the kinds of tasks you might do in practice: what knowledge is involved, and what expertise is involved? How easy are they to separate?

As we saw in Chapter 1, social work theorists have argued from a range of different perspectives that the working practices of social work carry a transformative quality, whereby the application of knowledge from fields of psychology, sociology, social theory, human growth and development and so on, involves something happening 'on the ground', which is relational and contextual. Social work is a 'practice', both in the sense that its proficiency arises from the rehearsing and repetition of activities until they are mastered, and in the sense that such rehearsing and repetition occur within the *application* of knowledge, rather than knowledge by itself. The very fact that social work is a 'contingent non-linear task' of 'complex indeterminate work' (McBeath and Webb 2002: 1018) means that its expertise is structured, at least in part, by its situated locality. Indeed, it could well be argued that without a clearly detailed and agreed upon definition of what social work expertise *is*, and without an agreed set of theoretical perspectives to situate such a definition – why, in Fook's words, 'for social workers the whole idea of professionalism is contested territory' (2002: 26) – then the most ready-to-hand resource for social workers to *define* what they do is, quite simply, to *describe* what they actually do. But this leaves open the political question of how inevitable such descriptions are, and the philosophical question over the conditions by which practice is *spatialized* in this way: in short, how the boundaries of expertise are drawn. As Roger Smith argues:

> in order to achieve a holistic approach to practice, social workers must first bring an appreciation of their own structural location and the associated 'baggage' which exercises significant influence on both the opportunities available to them and the constraints which they experience. The place which the social worker occupies and the perceptions associated with this are thus implicated in all aspects of practice. (Smith 2008: 193)

If social work expertise requires a ground, then what – if we can risk a philosophical question *par excellence* – is the ground of this ground? In many senses, the preceding chapters have discussed different forms of Smith's 'baggage' that make up a number of different dimensions to this sense of situated locality – the *ground on which* interpretations are formed – as a core of social work knowledge. Whether it is the formal question of jurisdictional basis (see Chapter 4), the need to 'know where I stand' in order to identify the self-in-training (see Chapter 6), the space within which we relate to others as a community (Chapter 2), the insistence on the 'locality' of social work in a globalised world (see Chapter 7), or the effective-historical horizon through which we engage and understand others (Chapters 1 and 3), practice is premised on a physical or representative *locus* – that is, a tactile or material web of spatial relations (see Lash 1999: 7) – from which social work and philosophy speak to each other.

The debate over the nature of social work expertise is, likewise, invested in marking out some kind of locus as distinct or authoritative, which grounds the application of knowledge within social work contexts. However, this point may seem so obvious that it is frequently passed over for scrutiny, in favour of the more 'practical' questions: that is, they ask what specific models, frameworks or approaches fill in this locus? Yet, there are significant questions over how such a locus is *formed*, which emerge from a variety of perspectives. To take just a few examples:

1. For Webb, social work follows an epistemic process of practical knowledge-based actions (2001: 59). As we saw in Chapter 6, he places this in opposition to the drive for 'evidence-based practice' as the grounding for social work expertise: a drive, he argues, that is influenced by the idea 'that a formal rationality of practice based on scientific methods can produce a more effective and economically accountable means of service' (60). The problem, for Webb, is not 'evidence' per se, but the hierarchical structuring of positivist epistemologies which discredit the subjective and situated ways in which social workers make sense of the world. Thus, social work knowledge is *localised* through the sense in which the 'conceptual thinking' of a social worker is formed by the concrete demands of specific cases, targets and time management. That is, a social worker's thinking is based on heuristic evaluation – the short-cuts taken to make a decision, determined by the most salient features of the present – rather than an objectively reasoned appraisal of empirical evidence or controlled behaviours. Thus: 'it is the social worker's conception of how things are, rather than evidential facts *per se* which determine actions' (66). And Webb is far from alone in this appraisal: White *et al.*, for example, argue for the importance of 'practice-near research' to understand the effectiveness of policy implementation and practice standards, rather than relying on an evidence-base 'driven by a group of senior academics working closely with a small cadre of civil servants, and resistant to criticism from a very early point' (2009: 408).

    It is clear that such an insistence on locality stands in a problematic relation to the kind of knowledge that is certified by its evidence-base, which implies – through the checks and balances of research protocols – it is knowledge which transcends situations, and licenses a 'universal' application. To what extent does this presume a solid ground upon which to identify the actions and decisions of the social worker as 'social work' expertise (as opposed to, say, the 'common sense' that Maidment and Egan (2004) explicitly dismiss from the locus of practitioner skills)? In some cases, the boundary between the ideals of policy and the realities of practice is distinct; but can we always clearly define such a locality of practice, so that we are 'near' enough to the *right* thing?

2. The complementary line of thought is that the locus of practice should be the client's interests and needs. Irene Levin notes how 'the phrase – "begin where the client is" – nearly has the status of a key mantra in social work'; but notes also that the actual meaning of this 'where' is ambiguous – whether, for example, it means starting from where the client physically is, or emotionally is, or whether it is a thematic location (the client 'sets the agenda', so to speak), or something else (Levin 2009: 7–8). The same questions for the first locus above apply to this as well: how are we drawing this boundary – especially given that

the interpellative practice of naming someone a 'client' has already displaced them, in at least some sense, into a system not of their making (as was discussed in Chapters 3 and 5)?
3. 'Given that social work is expanding its influence into nearly every social institution' Charles Cowger once wrote, 'it is not surprising that its knowledge is diverse, lacks unity, and has significant gaps' (1994: 263). Whether this should be lamented, or unified and boundaried by a clear 'answer' to the profession's 'purpose and knowledge base', remains contested. Certainly, for Cowger, a single unifying metaphor – such as the 'strengths perspective' he discusses specifically – may be appealing, but the profession is 'simply too diverse' for this to work. And there is nothing new in this assessment: Flexner's famous report of 1915 on whether social work should be considered a profession or not noted that 'lack of specificity in aim affects seriously the problem of training social workers', because 'the occupations of social workers are so numerous and diverse that no compact, purposefully organized educational discipline is feasible' (Flexner 1915: 23). Cowger instead looks to useful 'alternative' perspectives; in his case, the strengths perspective. But does this, in itself, presume a degree of autonomy to the profession – to choose from a range of alternative knowledges and expertise – which has been contested on many fronts throughout the history of social work? On what ground is this interpretation made?
4. Abbott (1995), meanwhile, situates social work knowledge as a kind of *mediator* – a discipline whose purpose and function is to make connections across other disciplines, applied or theoretical. He therefore sees social work as taking the form of an 'advisory jurisdiction', which links together the jurisdictions of other professions. The knowledge of social work is, thus, the interpretation and modification of those boundaries of knowledge that separate different spheres of practice. This is, Abbott suggests, the 'social' aspect of social work. But on what *basis* should such advisory jurisdiction be listened to? And how does this sense of professional knowledge as mediation relate to the *immediacy* of the demands of practice?

Thinking through Practice

These questions are obviously not rhetorical. How would you answer the points raised here about the 'ground' of social work expertise?

Professional boundaries

As with the debates within the previous discussions, our concern here is with the 'why', rather than the 'how' of such a ground or locus. This is not to ignore the 'how': after all, there is no point trying to articulate a locus of practice, if nothing practical is going to take place within it. But the first step towards finding a realisable and effective 'how' answer, is to explore the ways in which the formation of this locus itself sets the parameters for effective practice: in short, why some things seem 'useful' to social work, and others don't.

Clearly, social workers tend to work within geographically 'local' areas, whether these are defined in terms of specific 'communities' or the boundaries of local government or service provision. But the boundaries that mark out social work as a 'local' activity are not simply geographical; not just because the work the social worker does is inherently interconnected to other territories of practice – shaped and affected by decisions made elsewhere, from local government level all the way up to the international financial markets – but also because the ways in which social work is 'localised' involve a negotiation of practice, expertise and the idea of social work as a profession. Dominelli (1997) has argued that, historically, social work's origins have meant that practice is always dependent upon higher authorities for its resources; whether these were Victorian philanthropists, the State, or – increasingly so – the consumer market. In each case, social workers have been required to demonstrate credentials appropriate to such authority: the moral worth of the early social work agendas; the need to demonstrate a clear sense of clientele, knowledge of them as a distinct group, and the rigour of its intervention methods and training procedures. In this sense, expertise is clearly related to the professional status of social work: they both provide, through a set of interrelated operations, a boundary around specific practices and understandings that constitute an exclusive occupation.

Bourdieu notes that the title of 'professional' is a 'symbolic capital that is socially and [...] legally guaranteed'; and that it is the 'symbolic scarcity of the title in the space of names of professions that tends to govern the rewards of the profession' (1991: 242) rather than the actual activities the professional carries out. In this sense, the expertise of the professional social worker has reflected the shift that Max Weber schematised in his 'iron cage' thesis: that the value of knowledge shifted within Western modernity from the traditional, situated forms of authority to the 'legal-rational' authority which governs industrialised modernity (which we discussed in both Chapters 5 and 6). For example, Kornbeck's model for the social work profession (1998) suggests that a series of points of exclusivity mark out the social worker from the non-professional: only licensed social workers can perform specialised tasks; such tasks are subject to commodification, rather than acts of unpaid charity; such licensing involves an institutional registration; some minimal credentials are required to be a license holder; and these are based on a common core education and a unified set of rules for practitioners. True to Weber's model of legal-rational authority, the boundaries that mark out the 'professional', on this reading, are inherently bureaucratic; and the sense of 'locality' they invoke is concerned with the establishment of control points for flows of information, rather than customs, values and traditions embedded within a particular place. In this way, the professional practitioner lays claim to the expertise to practise *across* geographical boundaries, by virtue of nationally or internationally recognised qualifications and licences. This, of course, ensures that standards of practice are clearly established, monitored and maintained. But for as long as social work has moved towards professionalisation – a process which is still contested and debated (see Payne 2000, 2006) – a counter-current has argued that the ideological basis of legal-rational 'professionalism' is contrary to the actual activities of social work practice itself. There is a sense in which the nature of social work as a contextual, relational practice resists the exclusivity of professionalisation, and embeds itself in 'everyday' practices, beliefs and knowledge: as captured by Parton and O'Byrne's distinction between the 'technical-rational' and the 'practical-moral' approaches to practice (2000: 30–1), which expresses a familiar dichotomy across the literature (see Welbourne 2009: 22). In particular, the top-down model of professional care provision which privileges certain kinds of knowledge over and above others: knowledge which served certain models of government and state control (see, for example, Tsui 2004), and devalued other possible models of expertise rooted in the 'ground-level' workings of everyday wisdom, community-focused interpretation and user-based alternatives. In this way, the formation of professional expertise thus sits within longstanding tensions between knowledge and locality, and theory and practice. Younghusband (1951), for example, famously argued that the influx of journal articles parading high theory and inventing neologisms was a necessary evil of professionalisation: the language of the professions was the language of the scholar, not the practitioner (perhaps used to obtain 'conversion to a higher order of thinking, rather than to assist in transforming [...] practice.' (Fook 2002: 7)). Perhaps for this reason, in some countries at least, social work's relationship with the culture of the intellectual has historically been awkward and often suspicious (see Jones 1996): in overly-simple terms, the practitioner is *not* an intellectual, and therefore must *know* something the intellectual does not.[1]

The way in which the definition of social work expertise becomes a territorialising act in this way demands some further analysis. On Parton and O'Byrne's technical–rational model, professionalism and expertise are linked to formal scientific knowledge. Knowledge is based on accredited authorities; publicly accessible, written, evidence based, and testable. Professional practice, therefore, follows something of a 'diagnosis and treatment' model. A case is compared to existing explanations for its similarity, and once its description finds a match, an assessment can be made. Just as with Martin Davies's 'maintenance approach' (1985), this is a profession that works at the level of individual intervention: facilitating care rather than attempting to change the direction of an entire society. For the practical–moral model, meanwhile, personal excellence or worth, and the ability to promote healing through personal intervention, are the markers of the professional: emotional engagement and normative judgement within cases are seen as a core aspect of social work, leading to 'a broader approach that encompasses practical reasoning, emotion and, most of all, an intelligence that is disciplined and creative' (Taylor and White, 2001: 951). Resonating with the emancipatory approaches of critical and radical social work (Dominelli 1997), such a model emphasises the inter-relationality of everyday experience as the core of social work expertise: and the practical knowledge of how these relations occur means a strictly individualist approach is impossible. The social worker helps the marginalised to *understand* their social reality, and therefore change it: which involves bridging the service user's experience with the wider social issues that shape it.[2]

Our concern here is not to re-tread the debate over the merits of either side (or the dichotomy itself), but rather the way in which these two approaches articulate the locus of practice in different ways. Healy points out that the 'dominant discourses' governing the technical–rational approach, broadly construed – biomedicine, economics and law – are all 'strongly aligned with Enlightenment ideals of objectivity, rationality, individualism and linear notions of progress. In many health and welfare institutions, these discourses profoundly influence what counts as true, right and rational ways of proceeding' (Healy 2005: 18; see Thyer 2009) For example, in the context of clinical social work in the US, Irving and Young write that:

> Social work education and practice is still bound to the rigidities of an Enlightenment aesthetic with its entrapments of instrumental reason, and its conceptual arrangements of knowledge as hardened totalities and universal objectivity, an aesthetic where all differences have faded into a monochrome that blots out diversities. (2004: 216)

As we saw in Chapter 6, such values play down the significance of physical and interpretative location to our applied reasoning. Through such rigidities – for example, the condemnation of 'prejudice' as detrimental to knowledge – the engaged interpretative horizons that are the core of any profession's expertise (but, as our examples above showed, are particularly visible within social work) can be obscured. But more than this, it can arguably also create a distinct space, set apart from the everyday contexts in which social work comes into effect. In Michel de Certeau's words, such models of expertise:

> all postulate the constitution of a space of their own (a scientific space or a blank page to be written on), independent of speakers and circumstances, in which they can construct a system based on rules ensuring the system's production, repetition and verification. (1984: 24)

This is in many senses another way of articulating the space of the 'scientific method': which requires demarcating a place, defined by its own self-regulating procedures (falsification, rational objectification and so on), that forces a division between the everyday world or practice from the domain of 'proper' expertise. The world as we live it is reconstructed according to rules for how best to live. For de Certeau, 'this cleavage organises modernity. It cuts it up into scientific and dominant islands set off against the background of practical "resistances" and symbolizations that cannot be reduced to thought' (1984: 6). No surprise, then, that such discourses are accused of seeming too detached and abstracted from the roots of social problems that social workers deal with; and, likewise, the collection of professional 'traits' they demand (see Wiles 2013) can seem ill-fitting for the participatory and supporting practices in the field (Healy 2005: 19). Fook (2004) notes that, while discourses of professionalism based on traits or status may vary, they both share the sense that professionalism involves a knowledge dimension, a value dimension and a control dimension. For de Certeau, these are all rooted in a particular strategic formation of space in which professional practice emerges.³

But conversely, there is a serious problem for the practical–moral approach; and, indeed, the location of expertise within 'grounded' or 'engaged' practice rather than 'objective' reasoning: how does it draw a boundary around the *particular* lived experience of the 'everyday', in order to shape the locus of 'practice wisdom' which defines the professional expertise of the social worker?

Phronesis, interpretation and location

Philosophically, the concept of practice wisdom has its roots in the Aristotelian concept of *phronesis*. *Phronesis* – the wisdom of practicality – was, for Aristotle, the most important of the intellectual virtues, as it was needed to manage both *epistemē* (knowledge in its universal form) and *technē* (the technical knowledge of how things work). For example, consider a social worker involved with a group of young people, on a project about raising their self-awareness and employability. In such a situation, the worker will have knowledge of the outcome they want, and an awareness of the resources and materials available to them. This reflects, on Aristotle's distinction, the *epistemē* (the knowledge of what makes someone more employable; the wider sense of the importance of employment as an aspect of social capital; the enhancement of prospects and so on), and the *technē* (the technical capacity to use a PowerPoint presentation etc.). But these by themselves won't make the activities the worker does successful. They need to know how to act within concrete situations, and how to utilise the resources around them in order to achieve the ends they are aiming for. This 'knowhow' is *phronesis*, which, Aristotle argues, 'is concerned with things human and things about which it is possible to deliberate; for […] no one deliberates about things that cannot be otherwise, nor about things which have not an end [that is, an aim or purpose], and that a good that can be brought about by action' (1141b 8–12). The idea of 'knowhow' is thus a negotiation of technique and epistemology in an applied context.

This basic sense of *phronesis* seems to articulate the mediating techniques that Abbott wrote of above, as well as the heuristic and embodied knowing that Webb described. It is a distinctive kind of expertise: not quite the *epistemē* of the universal knowledge (a modern form of which is demanded by Kornbeck's model of professionalism), or the instrumental techniques of the labourer. In this way, *phronesis* is not practice in itself, but an interpretative relationship between the components of practice: the kind of knowhow which becomes visible as a form of expertise 'only at moments of confrontation when something significant is at stake' (Frank 2012: 64). Hence, in the context of assessment training, Whittington argues that 'learning that is restricted to technical competence renders the social worker more bureaucrat than professional and creates over-dependence on the perspectives of the authors of technical assessment tools' (2007: 18). The issue is not purely epistemological, though. It is based on the concrete reality of interpretative practice: a purely 'technical' approach to assessment may restrict 'the social worker's ability to recognise and question a conservative or illiberal assessment tool [...] with corresponding limits on his or her capacity to represent the interest of the service user' (18; see also Prescott 2013).

While it is true that '*having phronesis* is iteratively dependent on *practising phronesis*', (Frank 2012: 48, my emphasis), practical wisdom is not simply the expression of the practical demands of a given situation. *Phronesis* arises from, and is perpetuated by, histories of making sense of the world, and the practices which enable and limit such a sense-making. Hence, while it can be argued that social workers 'have a unique, up-close and personal perspective on social problems, their causes, their effects, and the role of policy in ameliorating or exacerbating them' (Hrostowski 2013: 50), this 'up-closeness' *by itself* does not constitute wisdom. Aristotle reminds us that 'practical wisdom [...] must be a reasoned and true state of capacity to act with regard to human goods' (1140b 20–1). *Phronesis* is not concerned with the primacy of common sense or unquestioned habits: it is applied wisdom, but still wisdom nonetheless, and as such is not opposed to method or theory *per se* (Landman 2012: 27). As wisdom, it articulates knowledge and reasoning that go well beyond the immediacies of day-to-day life and into the working conditions and structures that give our lives meaning. Indeed, the risk in over-emphasising the 'practical' aspect of social work – focusing on field education or placement-based learning as the distinctive feature of what is learned in social work education, for example – is that we ignore broader practices of socialisation which 'facilitate the integration of theory and practice and that support the development of the emerging professional for competency' (Earls Larrison and Korr 2013: 197–8). These are also aspects of *phronesis*: the key to practical expertise is not its opposition to the *episteme* of 'theory', but rather the building of a set of dispositions which shape the professional's interpretation of a case. The locus which *phronesis* demands is (at least on Aristotle's view) both spatial and moral.[4]

There is a danger of this becoming circular, though. If 'practice' is action regarding human goods, and human goods are constituted by their practice, then the very real danger is that *phronesis* drops back into a simple claim to local*ism*: that is, an unreflective sense of 'what we've always done here' which remains antagonistic to any pollutants from 'outside' that locality – be they theories, practices or directives. As Sheldon once wrote in defence of scientific principles within social work, 'collective mind sets and an unwillingness to debate complicated propositions have always got us into trouble in the past' (2001: 803). There is a risk that invoking a moral 'we' can reproduce an insular politics of location (see Chapter 3).

Furthermore, such a risk is clearly heightened by the *lack* of the clear sense of a coherent 'practising community' which the ancient account of *phronesis* relied on: as we discussed in Chapter 2, this can lead to reductive or simplified projections of communal identity which obscure any subordination or marginalisation of its members. For Aristotle, the moral direction of *phronesis* was structured around the need for a community to reach the goal of 'flourishing'; but the fact that his specific term for this goal is *eudaimonia*, literally translated as 'well-Goddedness', shows how awkwardly this translates into contemporary parlance. Indeed, as we saw in Charles Taylor's arguments explored in Chapter 6, the modern sense of 'flourishing' can frequently fall into disengaged and individualistic ideas, whether in the form of inner wellbeing or financial cost-effectiveness. And on a pragmatic level, the further risk of this localism is that it ignores the ways in which locality serves a strategic role in the distribution of social care: the fact that the frontline of practice is, necessarily, localised, can ignore the way in which the border of this frontline is often constructed from far afield, and shaped by directives and budgets decreed from a broader locale.

Thinking through Practice

How many of the problems raised for the Aristotelian concept of *phronesis* are also problems for the practical–moral approach to social work, as you understand it? What do you think the main differences might be between them, when translated from Ancient philosophy to contemporary practice?

Expertise and local knowledge: everyday tactics

One perspective that can be applied to such problems is Michel de Certeau's body of work, which inquires specifically into the formation of 'expertise' in terms of the relationship between knowledge, culture and location within contemporary society.

He introduces his concerns about how the relationships between general cultural practices and specific knowledge are affected by modern spatializing practices with reference to two figures: the 'Expert' and the 'Philosopher'. The Expert – who seems to resemble the Weberian professional outlined earlier – is a specialist, who is tasked with introducing their specialist knowledge into 'the more complex area of socio-political decisions' (1984: 6–7). The Philosopher – who bears more of a resemblance to Aristotle's bearer of practical wisdom – is, conversely, tasked with raising general questions, often sceptically, of specific techniques. More and more in contemporary society, de Certeau suggests, the Expert appears to 'blot out' the Philosopher. While both mediate between 'society and a particular body of knowledge' (6), the current value of knowledge is situated within the 'applied' (the domain of the Expert), and not the 'general' (that of the Philosopher).[5] Whereas, for Aristotle, the specialist techniques of practice (*technē*) were instrumental means to achieve a goal established by the wider *episteme*, de Certeau argues that now 'competence is transmuted into social authority'; an authority which is premised on the ability of the Expert to translate their specialist competences into other fields (or, in the case of social work, to demonstrate its 'value' to other professions, its 'usefulness' to the society it serves, its 'cost-effectiveness' within budgets, etc.).

However, the success of the Expert:

> is not so terribly spectacular. In him [*sic*], the productivist law that requires a specific assignment (the condition of efficiency) and the social law that requires circulation (the form of exchange) enter into contradiction. […] the Experts intervene 'in the name of' – but outside of – their particular experience […] through a curious operation which 'converts' competence into authority. […] Ultimately, the more authority the Expert has, the less competence he has. (7)

Because mere technique is not enough to warrant authority beyond each job it is applied to, the Expert cannot gain social authority from it; and instead, the expert assumes authority by virtue of *the place from where he speaks*. At this point, once Expertise is grounded in a separate, distinct place, it becomes unclear (for de Certeau) whether such a place is formed from a specialist knowledge, or from the dominant socio-economic ordering of society. This leads, as Nana Last explains, to a state where 'the production of expertise cannot but produce an unsustainable autonomy, one that ironically confuses what knowledge comes from "within" a discipline and what comes from that which is defined as the outside' (Last 2008: 15). Ultimately, the Expert can no longer know whether they are saying something specialised, or simply rehearsing the values of the general order of society. And it is at this point, de Certeau suggests, that 'their discourse is seen to have been no more than the ordinary language of tactical games between economic powers and symbolic authorities' (8).

De Certeau's account of the Expert is only a preliminary set of brush strokes for his larger study; and not meant to be utterly analogous to the question of social work expertise (although parallels can be made). For our purposes, it is a way of unpacking how any delineation of a locus of expertise is not simply a question of content, but also one of spatial structure. Key to the domination of particular forms of knowledge that define and shape 'professional expertise' is, de Certeau argues, the way in which the '*temporal* articulation of places' is transformed into a '*spatial* sequence of points' through the use of either 'strategies' or 'tactics' (1984: 35).

For de Certeau, traditional philosophy and social science – not to mention social policy and governmental agenda – have focused on strategies of space, and as such have seen this kind of rationalisation as a one-way street (think of Adorno's view of the culture industry in Chapter 7, which emphasised distinctive facets of our 'real lives' in order to order and regulate our activities). Because of this, the 'everyday' and the 'ordinary' are traditionally *spoken for* by the strategists: in all of the great social thinkers – Marx, Weber, Foucault, Bourdieu and so on – there is a tendency, de Certeau suggests, to see the everyday as a passive sphere of acceptance (although some theorists are more attentive to this than others), which is only able to speak through the governing discourses of the ruling authorities. In this way, particular models of knowledge, knowing and becoming-expert translate into strategic organisations of space. He argues:

> the calculation (or manipulation) of [those] power relationships that becomes possible as soon as a subject with will and power (a business, an army, a city, a scientific institution) can be isolated. It postulates a *place* that can be delimited as its own and serve as the base from which relations with an *exteriority* composed of targets or threats (customers, competitors, enemies, the country surrounding the city, objectives and objects of research, etc.) can be managed. As in management, every 'strategic' rationalization seeks first of all to distinguish its 'own' place, that is, the place of its own power and will, from an 'environment.' A Cartesian attitude, if you wish [...]
>
> It would be legitimate to define the power of knowledge by this ability to transform the uncertainties of history into readable spaces. But it would be more correct to recognise in these strategies a *specific type* of knowledge, one sustained and determined by *the power to provide oneself with one's own place*. It makes this knowledge possible and at the same time determines its characteristics. It produces itself in and through this knowledge. (de Certeau 1984: 35–6, my emphasis)

There are two points of particular interest here. First, the way in which a locus of expertise is made 'readable' – that is, articulated and defined according to the demands placed on a 'dependent profession' – carries with it a commitment to a certain form of knowledge; the same knowledge that allows the kind of fragmentation and atomisation of social activity into clearly boundaried and hierarchical organisation. In the case of professional expertise, such strategies enact a break between the 'place' of social work and its other (i.e. whatever is 'not social work'), as well as erecting a boundary between 'professional' and 'everyday'. The strategy of the professional is a 'mastery of place through sight': by spatializing 'expertise', strategies allow foreign or outside objects to be observed, measured and absorbed into the expert's scope of vision. Strategies are technocratic: they are able to 'produce, tabulate, and impose these spaces, [and] when those operations take place' (30). But de Certeau argues that for all coercive and disciplinary techniques used by the dominant socio-economic order, participants within such an order are not passive.

Secondly, then, there is a sense in which this spatialising logic deceives itself, by assuming that the everyday use of its discourses and structures must follow it by the book. But as de Certeau shows through a number of studies of particular cultural activities, participants (who, for de Certeau, are consumers of and within culture and society, broadly construed) create 'networks of antidiscipline' (1984: xv) as a matter of everyday living, which *tactically* challenge the strategies imposed on them. Such tactics are no less calculated than strategies, but are actions 'determined by the *absence* of a proper locus' (37, my emphasis). Tactics, thus, do not obey the 'law of place'. In short, the very notion of 'locus', in the strategic sense, is problematised precisely by its *use*.

> **Thinking through Practice**
>
> Smith et al. (2012) note how de Certeau's ideas present a useful model for characterising service users' involvement with social workers, whereby their acceptance of the need for social workers to be involved in their lives 'is not a passive acceptance; it is negotiated in each encounter with a social worker'. Likewise, 'social workers rarely resist, in the sense of opposing, service user participation, but they practise it pragmatically and contextually in everyday contacts with clients' (Smith et al. 2012: 1473–4). In this sense, Smith et al. read 'the abstract and ill-defined meta-narrative of service user involvement' as a strategy whereby the locus of practice is defined by the 'proper' authorities (1473); whereas the pragmatic negotiation between social worker and service user operates through tactical interpretation and action.
>
> To what extent have you found service user engagement to be 'tactical', on de Certeau's description?

It is important to note that the terms 'strategy' and 'tactics' are schematic illustrations for de Certeau, rather than dualistic positions. They are ways of differentiating between ways of 'producing' and 'consuming' a locus of practice. De Certeau argues that social science traditionally fails to see the tactical use of culture because 'what is counted is *what* is used, not the *ways* of using' (1984: 35). Precisely because cultural use underlies 'discourse' and 'production' in this way, culture is *not* something that is 'authored', and not something that can be completely strategised (see de Certeau 1997). In other words, a focus on the production of goods, values, identities and meanings can obscure how they are interpreted and put to use to the ends of those who use them; much in the way that we saw, in Chapter 5, White et al. (2009) detail the ways in which social workers manipulated bureaucratic regimes; or Vicky White's account of the 'quiet resistance' by individual social workers to the ways in which protocols are circulated; or the complex collective movements of 'guerrilla' practices within the profession (see Turbett 2014).

In this way, de Certeau's definition of the culture of everyday life as a form of weaving relational meaning through the ordering practices of social institutions and organisations resonates with the notion of 'practice-near' social work expertise: both resist their practice becoming 'fragmented in order to be displayed, studied and "quoted" by a system which does to objects what it does to living beings' (1984: 26). At the same time, we must be careful not to fall into a simple dichotomy, whereby the 'reality' of lived experience replaces strategic theories. This is not simply because social work, as a 'dependent' profession, is always situated within particular strategies of space and place. It is also because insisting on the reality of 'practice' can, very quickly, become a further strategic demarcation of expertise: drawing a boundary and mapping a location of 'what counts' from what doesn't, just as the anti-theoretical dogma within certain social work practices have historically done. While resisting the language of technical–rational professionalisation, the logic remains. It is, perhaps, analogous to how discourses of 'empowerment' can themselves become power strategies (see Smith 2008: 38; see also McLaughlin 2008).

On the problematic need to find 'answers'

The issue with an appeal to practice–wisdom, then, philosophically at least, is not that it may be relativistic, localist, or anachronistic, but rather that it risks *becoming* all of these things when it implicitly assumes the *same spatial form* of locus of expertise as the technical–rational. That is: if practice–wisdom remains committed to a particular logic of spatial organisation, then it risks ending up as a descriptive, rather than interpretative, activity. This is perhaps another way of making the case that the questions raised earlier about the four different accounts of social work expertise suggested: that it is perhaps not the *content* of the facts, theories and knowledge that are the issue, so much as the relationship between the *requirement* of facts, theories and knowledge within practice, and the tactical employment of facts, theories and knowledge within the interpretative operations of social work.

I am reminded here of Harry Ferguson's critique of the radical social work tradition for its 'idealistic theoretical prescriptions of critical thinking', and the imbalance between the volume of their negative critiques ('don't be sexist, racist, classist and so on') compared to what they offer in terms of 'the actual practicalities of what *can* and often *should* be done' (2013: 119). Read in conjunction with de Certeau, I would argue that the problem here is not – contrary to how it may first seem – that there is *no* 'ground' for radical thought (that is, the idealism of the radical voice means that there is no sense of 'applied' practice, no shared consensus amongst practitioners, etc.). It is, rather, that the ground such an approach stands on is not fully articulated, in terms of who is speaking for what, about whom, when and why. This leads, for Ferguson, to the emergence of platitudes and superficial gestures towards social change that, in fact, *restrict* a deeper discussion: however grand its ambition, the locus it operates within is too limited, too small, and too 'localised'. Clearly, this is a counsel which should be heeded. But there is a corresponding risk to the ground of such critiques themselves. This is the expectation for theories of social work to be always providing a sense of *completion*; that is, to both critique *and* offer solutions; to engage with theoretical traditions *and* contemporary practice, *and* future directions *and* the critical past; to perhaps even see the resolution of the question of expertise as analogous, if not synonymous, with the resolution of frontline cases. In this sense, while a critique such as this challenges the political dimension of the 'usefulness' of social work theory, the risk is that it does not apply this same challenge *hermeneutically*: and if critique is meaningless without an 'answer', and if discussion is meaningless with a 'use', then we have already subscribed to a discourse of immanence whose answers have been laid out for us (in some cases, this subscription is made explicitly: see, for example, Lee 2014). This is the problem of the metaphysics of presence, which we discussed in Chapter 5. Even within the language of 'the realities of practice', there remains the possibility that a curiously inverted demand for a 'view from everywhere' arises, which implicitly presumes that transcending the world is necessary to examining it.

Thinking about the formation of the locus of expertise, rather than the specific content – and, in doing so, the way that the spatialising of such a locus can determine, to some extent, the content of the expertise itself – is one way of reassessing the nature and impact of demands for the 'practicality' of social work's engagement with other disciplines, and the kind of theories it employs. An emphasis on translating temporal relations into spatial location often underlies concepts of pragmatism and practicality, and continues to shape the manner by which social work expertise is located. Back in the 1990s, David Howe assigned this to the political direction of mainstream social work. Increasingly, he argued:

> [k]nowledge is used to help social workers collect appropriate information on clients as well as identify and classify them as particular types of service-user or problem-presenters. [...] Less and less is the social worker expected, or indeed allowed, to make an independent, on-the-spot judgement or diagnosis of what is the matter. Less and less is the social worker likely to respond with a tailor-made, professional intervention based on his or her own knowledge and skills. There is no requirement to explore the causes of behaviours and situations, only the demand that they be described, identified and classified.
> (Howe 1996: 91)

From a philosophical perspective, Gianni Vattimo has discussed how this notion that 'knowledge', in order to be deemed *proper* knowledge, is often ordered to be classificatory, typologised, and clearly delineated. These are forms of what he terms a 'politics of description'; a politics which perpetuates a particular set of beliefs and practices surrounding the nature of what truth is, what truth looks like and what command it has of the social world; a politics which 'is functional for the continued existence of a society of dominion, which pursues truth in the form of imposition (violence), conservation (realism), and triumph (history)' (Vattimo and Zabala 2011: 12). A politics of description insists on the inevitability of the present world, and the requirement of clarifying it according to particular principles of organisation. In this way, even with the changes to social work instigated by the personalisation agenda in the UK, for example, which was seen by some as a return to more traditional 'frontline' social work, the governing ideological values maintained a focus on individual 'facts' of a situation. This, in practice, means the domination of one, specific, strategising perspective (the 'budget-holder', the 'consumer', and so on) which guarantees the certainty of knowledge, over and above the complex interplay of perspectives, some of which are 'not yet framed' within the same logic of production (Vattimo and Zabala 2011: 138).

Hence, description and classification are privileged over and above interpretation and problematising not only as a result of technical–rational approaches to professionalism or political contexts of practice, but also the metaphysical structures –

what we referred to earlier as the 'ground of the ground' – on which these take place. It is in this way that, while Howe outlines the problem as one of focusing on conditions rather than causes, the search for 'causes' can itself *also* effectively become an act of classification by other means; particularly if the relationship between the theories of causation from social theory, sociology, psychology and the domain of practice are not articulated clearly. It is a similar problem to that which we find in Fook's reflection on the radical social work of the 1970s: whereby a 'rather large disparity between the expressed empowering ideals of the radical tradition, and how people lived and experienced it' (2002: 11) emerged, due to a form of 'moral and technical absolutism' that flew 'in the face of the intended traditional social work values'; largely due to the ill-fitting, outdated or overly-deterministic schemas (2002: 10). In this case, the attempt to explain one set of oppressive structures (marginalisation, poverty, exclusion) seemed to end up using another set (hierarchical separations of 'theory' and 'practice', gender disparities within education, etc.). While they write from very different contexts of 'practice', for both Fook and de Certeau, the question of expertise is a question of its way of use: the problem is not only epistemological, but also, more fundamentally, interpretative. And, as we saw in Chapter 1, this involves re-questioning a number of our assumptions about the categories we use ('self', 'culture', 'rights' and so on), as well as the effective histories which inform their place in our horizons.

It is perhaps not without irony that I quote Fook here, given her demand for more concrete accounts of how practice can achieve the values of social work, rather than rest with abstract theory, and the endless problematising of the social field it can lead to. In other words, Fook demands some *answers* that make sense within practice, rather than subjecting practice to the demands of hierarchically-structured 'theoretical' knowledge. For some readers, it may well be that the nature of this book, and the course it has attempted to steer, appear to be doing just the opposite. After all, where *are* the answers to these debates? Can philosophy *only* critique?

This would, I hope, mistake the use of abstraction as a form of *domination* – whereby philosophy tells social work 'how to think' – for the more humble approach, somewhat reminiscent of de Certeau's Philosopher, whereby some general questions are posed to a specific field of work, for the benefit of both the specific and the general. Thinking about how the concrete activities of good social work are grounded, and unpacking, however broadly, some of the debates in which the interpretative concerns of social work and philosophy resonate, does not in itself make the demands of practicality any *less* significant; but it may well help to articulate the nature of those demands more fully – so long as it is remembered that philosophy *alone* cannot provide 'answers' for practice, just as social work practice cannot solve problems of philosophy. Likewise, I hope to have shown that drawing on the rich history and experience of social work practice and research allows us to probe into the production of philosophy; and in this way, there is a hermeneutic circle between them which can continue to turn – and turn, I hope, meaningfully.

Notes

1   I think here of statements such as Brian Sheldon's (2001), that suggest critiques of evidence-based practice are made mostly by 'academics', but far less so by 'practitioners, managers or service users'. Such a rhetorical appeal to a commonplace identity as a defence against perceived theoretical posturing is not uncommon, but manages to create a paradoxical movement towards both an anecdotal, common-sense 'we' who can be identified and spoken for (a discrete form of interpellation), in order to argue for a evidence-based knowledge-base that undermines the strength of anecdote and common-sense.
2   The opposition between these positions is, of course, polemically caricatured; if the choice is limited to being between 'care managers or rationers of services' and making 'a positive contribution to the lives of poor and oppressed people' (Jones *et al.* 2004: 3). Even if few may still hold to Flexner's claim (1915) that the reward of the social worker lies in heaven rather than earth, applications to study social work on the basis of a conscious desire to 'ration care' are still in the minority; and, as Dominelli noted above (and Garrett echoed in Chapter 6), even the most conscientious statutory social work remains dependent upon the demands of wider socio-political structures. But the issue here is how the demands of professionalism shape the ground on which practice stands as a form of expertise.
3   A spatialising which, incidentally, also serves as a ground which facilitates what Fook and others have described as the deprofessionalisation of social work into fragmented working practices, short-term contracts and (see Fook 2004: 32).
4   The notion of 'applied *phronesis*' has found a popularity in certain areas of the social sciences (see Flyvbjerg 2001; Flyvbjerg, Landman and Schram 2012), as a method of synthesising concerns for social justice (through empirical analysis of gains and losses, advantages and disadvantages with a particular area) with the desire for social change (through the use of moral reasoning). For Landman, for example, Aristotle's claim that 'all knowledge and choice aims at some good' (1095a 15) provides contemporary *phronesis* the means to bring together the often distinct concepts of 'value' and 'rationality', by placing any practical situation under four specific questions: where are we going? Who gains and who loses, and by which mechanisms of power? Is this development desirable? What, if anything, should we do about it (Landman 2012: 36)?
5   Garrett (2013: 213–15) discusses this particular shift in the identification of 'useful knowledge' in terms of the role of social theory within social work provision in the UK; outside of social work itself, a large debate remains as to whether the Higher Education Funding Council for England (HEFCE) has safeguarded subjects within science and medicine while demanding arts, humanities and the social sciences prove how their work has demonstrable 'economic impacts', and the extent to which this reflects neoliberal or neoconservative policies regarding the funding of education (see Bailey and Freedman 2011; for a more global view, see Nussbaum 2012).

References

Abbott, A. (1995) 'Boundaries of Social Work or Social Work of Boundaries?' *Social Service Review*, 69, 545–62.

Aristotle (1984 [350 BCE]). 'Nicomachean Ethics.' W. Ross and J. Urmson (trans.), in Barnes, J. (ed.), *The Complete Works of Aristotle*. Princeton, NJ: Princeton University Press, pp.1729–867.

Bailey, M., and Freedman, D. (eds.) (2011). *The Assault on Universities: A Manifesto for Resistance*. London: Pluto Press.

Bourdieu, P. (1991). *Language and Symbolic Power*. G. Raymond and M. Adamson (trans.). Cambridge: Polity.

Cowger, C. (1994). 'Assessing Client Strengths: Assessment for Client Empowerment.' *Social Work*, 39, 3, 262–8.

Davies, M. (1985). *The Essential Social Worker: A Guide to Positive Practice*. 2nd edn. London: Heinemann.
De Certeau, M. (1984). *The Practice of Everyday Life*. S. Rendall (trans.). Berkeley, CA: University of California Press.
—— (1997). *Culture in the Plural*. T. Conley (trans.). Minneapolis, MN: University of Minnesota Press.
Dominelli, L. (1997). *Sociology for Social Work*. London: Macmillan.
Earls Larrison, T. and Korr, W. (2013). 'Does Social Work Have a Signature Pedagogy?' *Journal of Social Work Education*, 49, 2, 194–206.
Ferguson, H. (2013). 'Critical Best Practice.' In Gray, M. and Webb, S. (eds), *The New Politics of Social Work*. Basingstoke: Palgrave Macmillan, pp. 116–27.
Flexner, A. (1915). 'Is Social Work a Profession?' *Proceedings of the National Conference of Charities and Corrections*. Chicago, IL: Hildemann.
Flyvbjerg, B. (2001). *Making Social Science Matter: Why Social Inquiry Fails and How it can Succeed Again*. Cambridge: Cambridge University Press.
Flyvbjerg, B., Landman, T. and Schram, S. (eds.) (2012). *Real Social Science: Applied Phronesis*. Cambridge: Cambridge University Press.
Fook, J. (2002). *Social Work: Critical Theory and Practice*. London: Sage.
—— (2004). 'What Professionals Need from Research: Beyond Evidence-Based Practice.' In Smith, D. (ed.), *Social Work and Evidence-Based Practice*. Gateshead: Athenaeum Press, pp. 29–46.
Frank, A. (2012). 'The Feel for Power Games: Everyday Phronesis and Social Theory.' In Flyvbjerg, B., Landman, T. and Schram, S. (eds.), *Real Social Science: Applied Phronesis*. Cambridge: Cambridge University Press, pp. 48–65.
Garrett, P. (2013). *Social Work and Social Theory*. Bristol: Policy Press.
Healy, K. (2005). *Social Work Theories in Context: Creating Frameworks for Practice*. Basingstoke: Palgrave Macmillan.
Howe, D. (1996). 'Surface and Depth in Social-Work Practice.' In Parton, N. (ed.) *Social Theory, Social Change and Social Work*. London: Routledge, pp. 77–97
Hrostowski, S. (2013). 'Social Work: A Harbinger of a New Progressive Vision?' *Race, Gender & Class*, 20, 1, 49–55.
Irving, A. and Tomas Young, T. (2004). '"Perpetual Liminality": Re-Readings of Subjectivity and Diversity in Clinical Social Work Classrooms.' *Smith College Studies in Social Work*, 74, 2, 213–27.
Jones, C. (1996). 'Anti-Intellectualism and the Peculiarities of British Social Work Education.' In Parton, N. (ed.), *Social Theory, Social Change and Social Work*. London: Routledge, pp. 190–210.
Jones, C., Ferguson, I., Lavalette M. and Penketh, L. (2004). *Social Work and Social Justice: a Manifesto for a New Engaged Practice*. Available at: http://www.liv.ac.uk/sspsw/manifesto/Manifesto.htm
Kornbeck, J. (1998). 'Researching Social work Professionalisation in the Context of European Integration.' *Social Work in Europe*, 5, 3, 37–45.
Landman, T. (2012). 'Phronesis and Narrative Analysis.' In Flyvbjerg, B., Landman, T. and Schram, S. (eds.), *Real Social Science: Applied Phronesis*. Cambridge: Cambridge University Press, pp. 27–47.
Lash, S. (1999). *Another Modernity, a Different Rationality*. Oxford: Blackwell.
Last, N. (2008). *Wittgenstein's House: Language, Space, and Architecture*. New York: Fordham University Press.
Lee, C. (2014). 'Conservative Comforts: Some Philosophical Crumbs for Social Work.' *British Journal of Social Work*, 44, 2135–44.

Levin, I. (2009). 'Discourses Within and About Social Work.' *Journal of Comparative Social Work*, 1, 1–18.

Maidment, J. and Egan, R. (2004). *Practice Skills in Social Work and Welfare: More Than Just Common Sense*. London: Allen & Unwin.

McBeath, G. and Webb, S. (2002). 'Virtue Ethics and Social Work: Being Lucky, Realistic and Not Doing one's Duty.' *British Journal of Social Work*, 32, 1015–36.

McLaughlin, K. (2008). *Social Work, Politics and Society*. Bristol: Policy Press.

Nussbaum, M. (2012). *Not for Profit: Why Democracy needs the Humanities*. Princeton, NJ: Princeton University Press.

Parton, N. and O'Byrne, P. (2000). *Constructive Social Work: Towards a New Practice*. Basingstoke: Palgrave Macmillan.

Payne, M. (2000). *Anti-Bureaucratic Social Work*. Birmingham: Venture Press.

Payne, M. (2006). 'Identity Politics in Multiprofessional Teams Palliative Care Social Work.' *Journal of Social Work*, 6, 2, 137–50.

Prescott, D. (2013). 'Social Workers as "Experts" in the Family Court System: Is Evidence-Based Practice a Missing Link or Host-Created Knowledge?' *Journal of Evidence-Based Social Work*, 10, 466–81.

Sheldon, B. (2001). 'The Validity of Evidence-Based Practice in Social Work: A Reply to Stephen Webb.' *British Journal of Social Work*, 31, 801–9.

Smith, M., Gallagher, M., Wosu, H., Stewart, J., Cree, V., Hunter, S., Evans, S., Montgomery, C., Holiday, S. and Wilkinson, H. (2012). 'Engaging with Involuntary Service Users in Social Work: Findings from a Knowledge Exchange Project.' *British Journal of Social Work*, 42, 1460–77.

Smith, R. (2008). *Social Work and Power*. Basingstoke: Palgrave Macmillan.

Taylor, C. and White, S. (2001). 'Knowledge, Truth and Reflexivity: The Problem of Judgement in Social Work.' *Journal of Social Work*, 1, 1, 37–59.

Thyer, B. (2009). 'Evidence-Based Practice, Science and Social Work: An Overview.' In Roberts, A. (ed.), *Social Worker's Desk Reference*, 2nd edn. New York: Oxford University Press, 1115–19.

Tsui, M. (2004). 'The Supervisory Relationship of Chinese Social Workers in Hong Kong.' *The Clinical Supervisor*, 22, 2, 99–120.

Turbett, C. (2014). *Doing Radical Social Work*. Basingstoke: Palgrave Macmillan.

Vattimo, G. and Zabala, S. (2011). *Hermeneutic Communism: From Heidegger to Marx*. New York: Columbia University Press.

Webb, S. (2001). 'Some Considerations on the Validity of Evidence-based Practice in Social Work.' *British Journal of Social Work*, 31, 57–79.

Webb, S. (2009). 'Against Difference and Diversity in Social Work: The Case of Human Rights.' *International Journal of Social Welfare*, 18, 307–16.

Welbourne, P. (2009). 'Social Work: the Idea of a Profession and the Professional Project.' *Locus SOCI@L*, 3, 19–35.

White, S., Broadhurst, K., Wastell, D., Peckover, S., Hall, C. and Pithouse, A. (2009). 'Whither Practice-Near Research in the Modernization Programme? Policy Blunders in Children's Services.' *Journal of Social Work Practice*, 23, 4, 401–11.

White, V. (2009). 'Quiet Challenges? Professional Practice in Modern Social Work.' In Harris, J. and White V. (eds), *Modernising Social Work: Critical Considerations*. Bristol: Policy Press, 129–144.

Whittington, C. (2007). *Assessment in Social Work: A Guide for Learning and Teaching*. Social Care Institute for Excellence. Available at http://www.scie.org.uk/publications/guides/guide18/

Wiles, F. (2013). 'Not Easily Put into a Box: Constructing Professional Identity.' *Social Work Education*, 32, 7, 854–66.

Younghusband, E. (1951). *Social Work in Britain: A Supplementary Report on the Employment and Training of Social Workers*. Dunfermline: Carnegie United Kingdom Trust.

INDEX

Abbott, A. 175, 179
Adorno, T. 162–5, 182
Althusser, L. 109–10 *see also* Interpellation
Anderson, B. 39
applied wisdom 9, 33n2, 47, 130, 172, 177, 179–81, 185, 188n4
Aristotle 38, 49, 52, 93 179–81
Askeland, G. 154, 159–60

Badiou, A. 51, 89, 96–100, 162
Baines, D. 54, 56
Barnes, M. 72, 137
Baudrillard, J. 98, 155
Bhabha, H. 157, 160, 162, 167
Bourdieu, P. 45, 123, 176, 182
British Association of Social Workers (BASW) 85, 100
Brown, W. 43, 65, 70, 72, 156–7
bureaucracy 22, 106–8, 112, 118, 121–2, 157
Butler, J. 109–12, 121

Cartesianism *see* Descartes
casework 16, 27, 36, 49, 106, 127
de Certeau, M. 77n4, 157, 165, 178–9, 181–5, 187
Charities Organisation Society (COS) 5, 27, 127, 135
communitarianism 46, 49, 51–3, 56
community: as different from society 38–40; communitarian model of 46–50, 177, 180; as a form of culture 85, 88–9, 93, 154, 157, 161–2, 164, 166; definitions of 36–7; inoperative *see* Nancy, J-.L; liberal model of 40–6, 54; responsible for care 49–50; wellbeing of 7; working within 10, 14, 36, 52, 56, 60, 117, 173
control vs care 7, 60, 118–19, 132, 137, 177–8
correspondence theory of meaning 19, 73–4
Cowger, C. 175
Cranston, C. 86–7, 89, 95, 97
critical practice 19
critical social work 10, 71, 77, 115, 131, 135, 177
critical thinking 10, 84, 130, 132–4, 139, 141, 146, 185
cultural competence 41, 91, 151, 154, 156, 163–4
cultural identity 77n4, 85, 161–2, 167
culturalisation of politics 154–7, 162

Deleuze, G. 67, 98, 162
deontology 73, 90
deprofessionalisation of social work 188n3
Derrida, J. 28, 94, 98, 108, 113, 115–23
Descartes, R. 128, 138, 183
différance 116
Dominelli, L. 5, 10, 36, 61, 64, 81–3, 101, 152, 160–1, 176–7

Earls Larrison, T. and Korr, W. 130, 180
economic: interests 76, 88, 137, 174, 182; liberal 38–40, 60; rationality 43–4, 51, 135–6, 178, *see also* reasoning; relations 5, 142, 152 11, 49, 119, 139, 142, 152, 159, 165; resources 7, 68, 161
efficiency 7, 135, 159–60, 182

empirical: evidence 26, 60, 75, 147, 166, 174; experience 3, 6, 85
empiricism 29, 92, 114, 129, 131, 138, 140
ethics: philosophical 4, 46–7, 73; cross-cultural 87; social work 6, 85, 91, 93, 95–102, 106–8, 120, 128, 151, 155, 168; *see also* human rights
Etzioni, R. 49
evidence-based practice 18, 26, 122, 128, 147, 174
expertise: contested definitions of 172–5; practical 179–80; power and 66, 155, 159; professionalization and 176–9, 181–3

Fanon, F. 157, 160
Ferguson, H. 115, 185
Ferguson, I. 20, 65, 71, 113
Flexner, A. 175, 188n2
Folgheraiter, F. 18, 22–3
Fook, J. 2, 17, 22, 64–5, 74, 76, 114–15, 165, 173, 177–8, 187
Foucault, M. 4, 72, 93, 129, 182

Gadamer, H-G. 23–6, 28–9, 31–2, 69, 74, 129, 141, 145–6, 157, 165
Garrett, P. 1, 33n5, 45, 98, 107, 108, 121, 142
du Gay, P. 121
Giddens, A. 49, 152
globalisation 129, 152–3, 158–9
glocalisation 160
Gray, M. 1–2, 8, 16–17, 21–2, 29, 31, 54, 98, 165
Grimwood, T. 2, 8, 77n1

Habermas, J. 8, 28–32, 36, 62, 146
Haug, E. 90, 159, 168
Hayek, F. 43, 51
Healy, K 26–7, 65–6, 68–70, 114, 121, 178
Healy, L. 153, 159, 165, 167
hermeneutics: cultural 9–10, 108, 172, 164; hermeneutic circle 26–8; horizon 23–5, 28–32, 69, 73–6, 111, 117, 129, 135, 141, 173, 178, 187; of restoration 20–3; of suspicion 28–30; of trust 23–6, 165; *see also* interpretation
Hobbes, T. 44–5, 91–4
Houston, S. 29–30, 32, 33n5
Howe, D. 2, 186–7
Hugman, R. 5, 91, 97
human rights: as a form of morality 46; as historical 83–4, 91–5; as a form of social work ethics 81, 84, 96–102, 155; 'third generation' *see* Cranston, C; as Western 83, 85, 87–90, 168; universal declaration of 81–2, 95

Imre, R. 6, 99, 100
International Federation of Social Work (IFSW) 7, 81, 99, 152, 160
International Association of Schools of Social Work (IASSW) 81
interpellation 108–10, 120
interpretation: as a philosophical foundation 8–10, 18, 24–5, 28–9, 67, 71, 141, 145, 186; Catholic 92; cultural 28, 46–7, 115, 155, 165, 167, 173, 177; deconstructive *see* Derrida, J.; grounds of 175; and ideology 29–30, 32; instrumental sense of 18–19; reactive 74, 76; in social work 14–17, 20, 23, 26, 31, 70, 180; tactical 184; 'thin' sense of 18

Jameson, F. 54, 151, 163
Jardine, D. 25, 27
Johnson, L. and Munch, S. 154–5, 157, 163–5
Jones, C. 1–2. 28, 65, 177, 188n2

Kant, I. 3–5, 30, 129
Kirk, S. and Reid, W. 26
knowledge: application of 173–5, *see also* applied wisdom; culturally situated 23, 28–31, 36, 46, 62, 153–5, 160–1, 163, 180–1; and expertise 172; 'knowledge of' and 'knowledge' for 27; knowledge-economy 118; implicit 128, 183; objective 18, 25, 27, 128, 134–5, 152, 182, 186, *see also* evidence-based practice; perpectivism 66; social work 10, 17, 26, 61, 65–7, 71, 75, 130–1, 139, 144, 151, 168, 173, 178; technical 101, 112, 115, 177, 179; Western context of 113–14, 139, 158, 176
Kornbeck, J. 39, 50, 176, 179

Lash, S, 33n4, 128, 173
Levi-Strauss, C. 39
liberalism 43, 46, 51–3, 56, 68, 72, 90, 97, 157, 160–1
locality 38, 152, 161–2, 165, 173–4, 176–7, 180–1
Locke, J. 91, 93, 129, 137–8, 140–3

McBeath, G. 16, 47–9, 57n2, 132, 173
MacDonaldisation 159
MacIntyre, A. 40, 45–9, 52–3, 55, 73, 92, 121
McLaughlin, H. 8, 20, 66, 74
'maintenance approach' to social work 177
Mamdani 155–6 *see also* culturalisation of politics

Marx, K. 33n4, 136, 182
Marxist 28, 71, 128, 136, 148n7
Maslow, A. 45
metanarrative 129, 136, 146, 160, 184
Midgely, J. 159
modernity 30, 38, 72, 108, 128–9, 132–3, 135, 139, 158, 176, 178
Moules, N. 17–20

Nancy, J-L. 37–8, 40, 51–6, 89, 156
narrative 41, 47–8, 61, 65, 69, 74, 106, 122, 128, 165, 167–8 *see also* metanarrative
narrative identity 137, 140–4, 146, 147n.2
National Association of Social Workers (NASW) 106, 151
natural rights 92–5
neoliberalism 43–4, 49, 65, 129, 153
Nietzsche, F. 61–2, 67–74, 76–7, 134
Nozick, R. 40, 43

objectivity *see* knowledge
O'Byrne, P. 118, 128, 130, 139, 143, 177
Oliver, K. 74
orientalism 158, 164

Pagden, A. 85, 94–5, 101
Parton, N. 6, 118, 128, 130, 139, 143, 152, 177
Payne, M. 128, 154, 159–60, 177
personalisation 49, 60, 62, 73, 75, 127, 136–7, 145, 186
phronesis *see* applied wisdom
political: critique 16, 28, 30, 173; demands 7, 39, 52, 87, 95, 119, 147; difference between politics and the political 53–4, 156; discussion 63, 65, 77n3, 98, 181; identity 17, 62; practices 5, 37, 61, 90, 93, 96, 158, 166; philosophy 40–1, 45, 49, 86, 91–2, 127, 142; post-politics 53–6, 157; power 67, 73, 81, 83, 160, 162, 164; social work politics 11, 99, 131, 137, 185–6
postcolonialism 74, 119, 158–62
postmodernism 77, 96–8, 120, 137, 146
poststructuralism 117, 121
power: active and reactive 67–9, 72–3; and authority 53, 81, 92, 109–10, 183; colonial 159; disempowerment 61–4, 72–3, 75, 82, 156; distribution of 41, 48, 108, 137; empowerment 4, 7, 18, 46–7, 54, 93, 99, 120, 155, 185, 187; within interpretative practices 21, 27–8, 30, 32, 112, 121, 123, 163; structures of 56, 62, 94–5, 114–15, 136, 139, 142; postcolonial 158, 167; within professional social work identity 66, 70
practical wisdom *see* applied wisdom
Price, V. and Simpson, G. 6, 37–8, 47, 49, 60–2, 66, 71–2, 74, 76
Prince, K. 118, 121, 123
profession, social work as a 2, 17–18, 26–8, 66, 100–1, 130, 143, 147, 152, 172, 186
professional imperialism 159, 168
professionalisation 113, 135, 159, 176–7

Ranciere, J. 8, 51, 64, 77n3
Rawls, J. 40–8, 50–4, 62, 68, 96–7, 95
Reamer, F. 106, 117
reasoning: applied 167, 177–80; different types of 3–5, 7; within interpretation 30, 40, 44–5, 145; in human nature 92; instrumental 132, 135–6, 145, 167
reflective practice 19, 26–8, 107, 127, 146
relativism cultural 84, 91, 97–8, 142; moral 25, 142; postmodern 77
ressentiment: difference with resentment 68–9; Nietzsche's concept of 67–71; in social work 72–77
Ricoeur, P. 20–1, 33n3, 108, 111, 119
Ritzer, G. see *MacDonaldisation*
Rossiter, A. 6–8, 25

Said, E. 158, 160, 163–5
Sassen, S. 153
Scheler, M. 69
Schön, D. 5, 106
Schram, S 109, 111, 121, 129
Searle, J. 21–2
self-identity 127, 129, 138, 140, 146
service user perspectives 19, 23–4, 28–9, 45, 56, 61–4, 66–7, 70, 74–6, 96, 117, 122–3, 177
Sloterdijk, P. 7n2, 152
Smith, A. 68
Smith, R. 7, 25, 75, 173, 185
social work education: critical thinking in 132; development of 27; experiential 39; as a global market 160, 163–4; practice placements 4; principles of 10–11, 18, 101, 147, 167, 178, 180; role of reflection in 106, 127; the self within 129–30, 137–9, 141, 143, 145–7; *see also* cultural competence
social work practice: with adults 75, 111, 45; with children 7, 19, 22–3, 28, 30, 45, 47, 75, 105, 111, 118, 122–3, 165–7; with communities *see* community; with homeless people 8, 43; international 90, 159, 168; with learning disabilities 42, 50,

55, 60, 74; with young offenders 36, 47, 161; with young people 75–6, 179
society: aims and values of 5, 11, 43, 67–8, 73; global 90; modern 4, 30, 38–9, 94–6, 121, 128, 135, 163, 181, 186; organisation of 54, 85–6, 109, 145; pluralist 36, 41–2, 83, 166; pre-modern 92–4
Spivak, G. 74, 119, 158, 160, 162
state of nature 44–5, 93
strategies and tactics, difference between 182–5

Taylor, C. 10, 63, 87, 129, 131, 134–7, 139–46, 157, 167–8, 181
technology 16, 108, 153
'Third Way', the 49
Thompson, N. 5, 8
tolerance 61, 68, 90, 157
Tönnies, F. 38–40, 44, 55
tradition: anti-intellectual 1; approaches to social care 62, 75, 132; in communities 41, 47–51, 91, 151; in hermeneutics 23–6, 29–32, 36; indigenous 158, 161, 165, 167; Western 87–8, 102, 123 n.2, 129, 176
training 112, 123, 129–134, 137–9, 141–3, 146, 168, 173, 175–6

underclass 169n1
utilitarianism 40, 73, 90, 92

values: and culture 38, 54, 88, 95, 97, 121, 152, 163, 166, 178; 'is' vs 'ought' 18, 140, 143; and identity 138–9; reactive 67–70, 73; in social work 29, 61, 72, 81, 84, 96, 101, 113, 132, 155, 168, 186–7; *see also* ethics
valuing people policy 61, 65–6, 71–2, 74, 76
Vattimo, G. 1, 9, 28, 32, 114, 164, 186

Ward, G. 9–10, 27, 32, 45
Webb, S. 1–2, 8, 16–17, 21–2, 27, 31, 43, 47–9, 54, 57n2, 84, 95–102, 132, 141, 168, 173–4
Weber, M. 33n4, 106, 112, 148n7, 176, 181–2
Wehbi, S. 159
White, S. 16, 122, 174, 177, 184

Younghusband, E. 177

Zabala, S. 1, 28, 32, 114, 186
Žižek, S. 65, 68–9, 87–90, 95–7, 157

LEWD LOOKS